BARRON'S

NURSING SCHOOL ENTRANCE EXAMS

4TH EDITION

Corinne Grimes, R.N., Ph.D.
The University of Texas at Austin
School of Nursing, Austin Texas

Sandra Swick, R.N., B.C., Ed.D., C.M.S.R.N.
McLennan Community College
Waco, Texas

Rita Callahan, R.N., B.S.N., M.A., Ph.D.

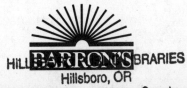

BARRON'S

All inquiries should be addressed to:
Barron's Educational Series, Inc.
250 Wireless Boulevard
Hauppauge, New York 11788
www.barronseduc.com

ISBN: 978-0-7641-4668-8

Library of Congress Catalog Card No. 2011019253

Library of Congress Cataloging-in-Publication Data
Grimes, Corinne.
    Barron's nursing school entrance exams. — 4th ed. / Corinne Grimes, Sandra Swick, Rita Callahan.
        p. cm.
    Includes index.
    Summary: "One multi-part model exam plus many shorter tests within each of this book's chapters
will give prospective nursing school applicants general orientation and solid preparation before they
take an actual nursing school entrance exam. While each entrance exam given by nursing schools
throughout the country will vary in topics covered, this manual offers comprehensive coverage of virtually all possible topics. Prospective nursing students will value the authors' detailed description of the
nursing profession, its duties, responsibilities, and satisfactions. That discussion is followed by a self-
assessment questionnaire to help readers decide if nursing is the right career choice for them. The
manual also provides test-taking strategies designed to enhance study skills and reasoning ability that
will be useful in any test situation. Also presented is a subject review that covers a range of testable
topics: verbal skill-building, reading comprehension, math, and science" — Provided by publisher.
    ISBN 978-0-7641-4668-8 (pbk.)
    1. Nursing schools—United States—Entrance examinations—Study guides. I. Swick, Sandra.
II. Callahan, Rita. III. Title. IV. Title: Nursing school entrance exams.
    RT79.G75 2011
    610.73076—dc23   2011019253

Printed in the United States of America

9 8 7 6 5 4 3 2 1

Contents

Introduction

CHAPTER 1

Is This Book For You?

Are you wondering what might be included on a nursing school entrance exam, or does the nursing program you've applied to require an entrance exam? If you answered yes to either of these questions, then *Nursing School Entrance Exams* is the reference you need.

Nursing school entrance examinations provide associate degree, diploma, and baccalaureate nursing programs with specific information relating to an applicant's or newly admitted individual's abilities in content areas that provide the foundation for nursing courses such as verbal ability, reading comprehension, numerical or mathematical ability, and life and/or physical sciences. Nursing school entrance examinations generally use a multiple-choice format.

Verbal ability includes elements such as vocabulary, antonyms, synonyms, verbal reasoning, and the use of analogy. Included in verbal ability are English usage and grammar, spelling, prefixes, suffixes, and root words.

Reading comprehension involves reading sentences, paragraphs, or short articles and answering questions, interpreting, and/or making inferences about the literary piece. Prior knowledge of the topic is not requisite for reading comprehension because the examination is asking you to think logically and make decisions based on the information presented.

Topics for verbal ability and reading comprehension may address technical or scientific knowledge and/or general, everyday knowledge. Information may come from discipline-specific vocabulary, English grammar, history, geography, literature, art and architecture, humanities, general information, natural sciences, social sciences, and mathematics.

Numerical ability encompasses arithmetic, fundamental algebra, and geometry. Computation and interpretation of word problems, charts, ratio and proportion, decimals, percentages, and fractions may also be included. Word problems, drawn from common life events, may address such areas as sales, taxation, insurance, distance or travel, geometry, age, mixtures, investments, interest, and averages.

The life and/or physical sciences section focuses on basic premises of biology, chemistry, human anatomy and physiology, health, and physics. Life sciences specifically addresses human structure and functioning, development, and genetics.

This book is intended to assist the individual to prepare or review for a nursing school entrance examination. This book is not intended to provide sufficient instruction on any topic in which one has little or no previous experience. For example, if you have never taken algebra or geometry, it is extremely doubtful that the algebra and geometry sections found in this book will provide a background that will enable you to be successful on similar sections of a nursing school entrance examination.

Nursing School Entrance Exams is not intended to address a specific nursing school entrance examination. Nursing programs using entrance exams have a number of examinations from which to choose. These standardized exams are used nationwide. A brief overview of selected nursing school entrance examinations is presented in the following table:

Overview of Selected Nursing School Entrance Examinations

Test	Content Areas	Number of Questions	Time Allowed (in minutes)
HESI A^2	Anatomy	50	50
	Basic Grammar	50	50
	Biology	25	25
	Chemistry	25	25
	Mathematics	50	50
	Reading Comprehension		50
	Vocabulary & General Knowledge	50	50
NET	Reading Comprehension	33	30
	Mathematics	60	60
	*(Reading Rate, Test-Taking Skills, Stress Level Profile, Social Interaction Profile, Learning Style)		
NLN PAX-RN	Mathematics		60
	Science		60
	Verbal Skills		60
PSB-RN	Part I: Vocabulary, Arithmetic, and Form Relationships (minitests)	30, 30, 30	30/minitest
	Part II: Spelling	50	
	Part III: Reading Comprehension	40	
	Part IV: Natural Science	90	
	Part V: Vocational Adjustment Index	90	
RNEE	Life Science	40	
	Numerical Ability	40	
	Physical Science	40	
	Reading Skill	45	
	Verbal Skill	50	
TEAS	English	55	65
	Mathematics	45	56
	Reading	40	50
	Science	30	38

*Does not count toward score

Features of This Book

The remainder of this introductory chapter provides basic information about the nursing profession and nursing programs available to individuals interested in becoming registered nurses in the United States. Information is also supplied regarding specialization versus generalist nurses, potential costs of a nursing education, financial assistance, nursing school entrance examinations in general, and graduate nursing education.

Chapter Two provides information and guidelines regarding general examination preparation and specific test-taking strategies regarding multiple-choice examinations.

There are separate chapters throughout this book that focus on verbal ability, reading comprehension, numerical ability, and science. Each chapter provides a basic review with related facts, concepts, and easily identifiable principles. Within each chapter are sample tests with answer sheets and answer keys with brief explanations or rationales for test items. The numerical ability sample test keys provide step-by-step solutions when more than one simple operation is required to obtain a correct answer.

At the end of the book is a multipart examination which provides an overview of all of the concepts and principles found in the book.

Nursing School Entrance Exams provides the essentials of what is needed to be successful on nursing school entrance examinations without pages of extraneous information.

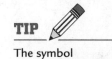

TIP

The symbol CHALLENGE appears before those practice questions that are more difficult than what you will be exposed to on an actual exam.

Nurses and What They Do

So you think you want to be a nurse. Nursing is one of the most gratifying careers you'll ever find. But nursing is not what you've seen on television soap operas or read about in books. Nursing is hard work, and learning to become a nurse requires dedication and long hours of study and preparation.

Unlike many other disciplines in which the academic curriculum has foundation courses with many related subject areas, nursing courses usually build on one another. The prerequisites courses, such as anatomy and physiology, chemistry, microbiology, and biology are key connections to understanding the actual nursing courses. The nursing program focuses on specific nursing courses and the application process. For example, it is expected that the nursing student comes to the nursing program with the ability to incorporate previously learned anatomy knowledge with newly acquired nursing knowledge and skills. When a pre-nursing student enrolls in prerequisite courses, it should be with the intention of seriously learning the information in transition to the nursing program.

Other prerequisites like English, history, and mathematics are equally pivotal in applying the learned knowledge in managing communication with patients, understanding how a patient's history is relevant to providing present care, and applying mathematics with precision, knowing that the medication you are about to administer to your patient is exact. Some pre-nursing students are grateful knowing they have passed a prerequisite course, perhaps wiping their forehead thinking, "I passed that one." The point conveyed is that each prerequisite is pre-empted to more comprehensive knowledge of the subject once admitted to the nursing program. As such, a weakness in one area may cause academic problems in the remainder of the nursing sequence. After all, advanced courses usually depend heavily on knowledge gained from prerequisites.

Today's nurses work in numerous roles and settings in our society. Opportunities are virtually unlimited. The following list includes settings in which nurses may practice:

Hospitals	Cruise ships
Clinics	Retirement/nursing homes
Doctors' offices	Volunteer organizations
Business/industry	Occupational health programs
Community agencies	Ambulatory care agencies
Schools	Hospices
Nursing schools	Private practice
Military	Federal/state agencies
Resorts and summer camps	

What a nurse actually does depends upon the practice setting. In the majority of institutional or home health settings, nurses provide care to individuals with chronic or acute physical and/or mental conditions. What a nurse does also depends upon the needs of the individual patient. The nurse may assume total care of a patient who is unable to meet any of his or her needs or may help only in areas where assistance is needed.

When working with patients, nurses assume a number of roles. In many cases, these roles overlap and are interdependent in nature. They include:

Caregiver	Role model
Comforter	Decision maker
Patient advocate and protector	Case manager
Teacher	Communicator
Counselor	Researcher

When practicing in these various roles, the nurse works to meet, or helps the patient meet, hygiene, elimination, safety, nutritional, spiritual, comfort, activity, sensory, adaptation, and/or mental health needs. The nurse focuses on assessing, analyzing, planning, and resolving actual or potential health problems and evaluates the effectiveness of nursing interventions based on the patient's responses.

Most people think of nurses as working with individuals on a one-to-one basis. In the community setting, however, the patient may not be an individual but a family or group of families, a group of individuals, or an entire community.

Educational preparation plays an important role in climbing the career ladder in nursing. Career opportunities run hand in hand with a nurse's educational preparation. Simply put, opportunities for advancement increase as education increases. For some levels of practice, an associate degree in nursing is acceptable. For others, a master's degree or a doctoral degree in nursing or education is required. Career opportunities include:

General duty or staff nurse

Private duty nurse

Home health nurse

Clinical nurse specialist

Nurse midwife

Nurse administrator

Nurse educator

Nurse researcher

Nurse consultant

Nurse anesthetist

Nurse practitioner

Is Nursing Right for Me?

Nursing is not for everyone, and it takes more than "desire" and a "big heart" to be a good nurse. Nursing requires intelligence, self-discipline, critical thinking, communication skills, compassion, dedication, high moral and ethical standards, endurance, as well as respect and concern for the welfare of others regardless of race, creed, culture, or religion.

In considering nursing as a career, think about the following questions.

☐ Is nursing a job or a career?

There is a difference between a job and a career. A job is something you do in exchange for something else, usually money, and nothing more. A career, on the other hand, is something you are dedicated to. A career is an endeavor in which you constantly strive to be the best at your craft and in which life-long learning is not only a necessity but a consuming desire.

☐ Am I a good team player?

In the majority of instances, nursing is a team effort focusing on an identified patient. No one person or specialty is more important than the other. The entire team must work together for the patient's welfare.

Broadly speaking, nurses are part of a team that includes a physician and other health care professionals. Depending upon the patient's needs, the team may also include case managers; physical, occupational, respiratory, enterostomal, and speech therapists; nutritionists; social workers; pharmacists; psychologists; and spiritual advisors. Narrowly speaking, the team is the group of health care individuals the nurse works with on a daily basis.

☐ Am I honest, dependable, responsible, and accountable?

These qualities are the hallmarks of a good nurse. Nurses must be honest in their relationships with patients and their families, physicians, and other health care workers. Nurses must also be honest with themselves and be able to seek appropriate assistance in situations in which they are not competent. Nurses must be dependable and come to work as scheduled and correctly perform their duties as prescribed. Nurses must also be responsible and accountable for their own behavior and actions. The patient, physician, or other health care workers cannot be blamed when nurses make mistakes.

❑ Do I engage in behaviors that have the potential to bring harm to myself, a patient, or others?

As a note of information, the majority of colleges of health science nursing programs are required by individual state boards of nursing, to conduct a criminal history background investigation of all nursing student applicants. Additionally, some schools require drug screens as well. Presently, all boards of nursing require fingerprinting for licensure. Health care employers require both background checks and drug screens.

Your clinical practicum is vital to learning nursing. You are provided didactic knowledge, and the clinical experiences allows for the application process of this learning. The numerous community healthcare facilities require verification of background checks prior to any nursing student entering their facility. The purpose for this is in the effort of ensuring safety and well-being of patients.

Nursing students are admitted conditionally, awaiting the results of the background check investigation. This background investigation is required during the first semester of admittance to a nursing program. Background checks for employment and school are separate. Results of your background check will be made available to you as the student and the appropriate nursing program of which you have registered.

Background checks are confidential. Some crimes are listed below and are considered crimes as examples. This list is not of an entirety of crimes:

- Assault and/or battery
- Homicide committed anytime
- Felony convictions
- Child abuse, sexual exploitation of children, child abduction, child neglect, contributing to the delinquency or neglect of a child, enticing a child for immoral purposes, exposing a minor
- Forgery and counterfeiting
- First- or second-degree arson
- Abuse, exploitation or neglect of a vulnerable adult (disabled or elderly) committed at any time
- Any charge related to illegal drugs such as (but not limited to) possession of drugs or paraphernalia
- Withheld judgments for felonies
- Poisoning
- Kidnapping
- Misdemeanor theft committed during the last 5 years
- Grand theft committed during the previous 7 years
- Delinquency or neglect or a child, enticing a child for immoral purposes, exposing a minor to pornography or other harmful materials, incest, or any other crime involving children as victims or participants committed at any time
- DUI within the last 3 years or more than one in the past 5 years
- Sexual assault, rape, indecent exposure, lewd and lascivious behavior, or any crime involving nonconsensual sexual conduct committed at any time

Drinking alcohol excessively, using illegal substances, abusing legal substances, and engaging in unprotected sex have the potential to bring harm to oneself and others.

Nurses whose judgment is chemically impaired risk harming themselves or, worse, a patient. Nurses with chemical dependencies are more likely to engage in illegal behaviors in order to meet the needs of their addiction and may report that certain medications were administered to a patient when in reality they gave the medication to themselves.

If you engage in any of these chemically related behaviors, you'd probably say that you'd never attempt to drive a car or care for a patient while in an impaired state, and you'd probably be telling the truth—to a point. The problem is that most individuals with chemically related problems do not realize when they are physically or mentally impaired.

Engaging in unprotected sex increases the risk of contracting HIV/AIDS that may be unknowingly transferred to patients and other sexual partners. Individuals exposed to HIV/AIDS may not show symptoms of the disease for months or years.

❏ Do I follow directions?

There is little nurses do that does not involve following directions of some sort. All health care agencies have policies and procedures that dictate proper behavior or actions to be taken with virtually any responsibility occurring within the institution. Nurses who take shortcuts or ignore institutional policies and procedures when performing patient-related tasks place themselves, patients, and others at risk for injury.

❏ Do I care for others?

Nurses do not selectively determine who they will care for. Nurses must administer to all regardless of gender, race, creed, culture, or religion. Nurses also do not selectively determine the quality of care that a patient is to receive. All patients deserve the highest standard of care possible.

❏ Am I comfortable with decisions others make even when I disagree with decisions they have made?

Individuals do not forfeit their constitutional rights or their ability to make decisions when they enter the health care system. Competent patients have the right to refuse any and all treatments without fear of reproach or retaliation, even if the end result will ultimately be death.

❏ How do I manage stress or crisis?

Nursing is a profession laden with stressful situations and ever-impending crises, be it patient or institution related. A patient's condition may suddenly worsen, or a nursing unit may have to work short staffed because of absenteeism. Nurses must have the ability to remain calm and collected during stressful or crisis situations in order to focus on the patient.

☐ How do I feel about death and dying?

Human life is fragile, and individuals entering the health care system sometimes die. The process of dying as well as death itself are normal parts of the human existence. An ancient Chinese proverb states "a child born is a child dying" because every minute of life is one minute closer to death. Death is a visitor to those too ill to recover, and death intervenes when all else fails. In order for nurses to work effectively with death and dying, they must understand and accept their own mortality.

☐ How do I handle frustration?

Caring for individuals in any health care setting can be frustrating and so is working with others. Patients may not be compliant with their medications or keep needed appointments. During a crisis, an institution may have difficulty in obtaining necessary resources. Nurses must be able to control their frustrations if they are to keep the patient's welfare in mind. Losing focus could bring harm to a patient or others.

☐ How do I respond to abusive behaviors?

Patients and their families are under great stress as a result of a serious illness and the possible need for hospitalization. As such, they may not always respond in a kind fashion. When patients are verbally abusive, they are usually striking out in frustration, grief, fear, pain, or anxiety. Oftentimes the nurse just happens to be the one to catch their wrath. For the nurse to be verbally abusive in return would be inappropriate and would make an already difficult situation even worse.

Physicians may be verbally abusive to nurses and other health care workers, or health care workers may vent their anger on each other. In all such cases, verbal abuse should not be tolerated.

Physical abuse should also not be tolerated and should be addressed according to institutional policy.

Selecting a Nursing Program

If you are seriously considering a career in nursing, you should realize that there is a difference in the types of nursing programs that can lead to a registered nurse designation. Each meets the needs of different types of students.

When selecting a school of nursing, it is important to consider the following questions.

What is the pass rate for the past five years of the school?

The pass rate is the percentage of graduates that have successfully completed the NCLEX-RN examination. Schools with consistently low pass rates over a number of years may have inadequately prepared faculty, new or outdated curriculum, or poor instructional methods. Some may have lowered their admission standards and therefore are graduating lower caliber students.

Is the school of nursing nationally accredited by a volunteer nursing agency or agency of higher education such as the National League for Nursing (NLN), American Nurses Association (ANA), the Commission on Collegiate Nursing Education (CCNE), or one of the associations of colleges and universities?

Accreditation from a national nursing agency is essential for admission to many graduate programs in nursing.

Is the school of nursing recognized by the state's Board of Nurse Examiners?

The board extends licensure to graduates who successfully write the NCLEX-RN and regulates the practice for registered nurses in a given state. The purpose of a state's Board of Nurse Examiners is to protect the public. It may suspend or remove an individual's license to practice nursing if that person is unable to meet the standards of practice for a given state.

What kind of reputation do graduates of the school of nursing have in the community or area?

If health care institutions had a preference, would they choose to hire graduates of one nursing school over another?

How good a fit would you be at a particular school of nursing or institution of higher education in which the school of nursing is located?

Do you prefer large educational institutions with a sizeable student population and numerous social and work opportunities, or do you prefer a smaller educational institution with a modest student population and fewer social and work opportunities? Larger institutions may offer more from a nonacademic standpoint. Smaller institutions may provide a close-knit community atmosphere and offer more personalized relationships with faculty and one-to-one assistance when necessary.

Do you need your own transportation to get to and from classes or clinical experience?

Schools of nursing typically do not furnish transportation to or from learning experiences on or off campus. Didactic or lecture courses are normally offered within the institutional setting. But clinical experience, that is, taking care of patients or clients in various health care settings, is usually conducted off campus, in some cases many miles away. There is also no guarantee that clinical sites will be within walking distance if the school of nursing is located in a large metropolitan area.

There are currently three avenues or programs to become a registered nurse in the United States. Each program has its specific educational foundation, type of curriculum, accrediting agencies, educational location, and professional organizations.

Associate degree programs are the shortest in length and usually require two years of nursing course work in addition to nonnursing subjects. Associate degree programs are often referred to as ADN programs and are usually found in community or junior colleges.

Students enrolled in ADN programs are required to take the general education courses all states require of college graduates. These include courses in English, history, psychology, literature or humanities, math, and general sciences. Required nonnursing courses may include anatomy and physiology, chemistry, nutrition, algebra, and microbiology. Associate degree nursing courses usually include nursing fundamentals, medical surgical nursing, mental health nursing, pediatric nursing, obstetric nursing, and history and issues in nursing. Critical thinking, ethical decision making, and problem solving are integrated into all nursing courses.

The second type of nursing program, *diploma programs*, are affiliated with hospitals and are usually three years in length. Diploma programs do not lead to an associate or baccalaureate degree so general education courses may not be required. Diploma programs do, however, require prerequisite courses. These may include anatomy and physiology, microbiology, nutrition, pharmacology, and psychology.

Nursing programs leading to a *baccalaureate degree*, the last type of program, are at least four years in length. These programs are located in four-year colleges, universities, university-affiliated medical centers, and health sciences centers. Like associate degree students, baccalaureate students are required to take the college's or university's general education requirements. Nonnursing or prerequisite courses may include anatomy and physiology, microbiology, chemistry, literature, fine arts, nutrition, ethics, logic, statistics, sociology, and psychology.

Nursing courses in baccalaureate programs typically include fundamentals of nursing; health and physical assessment; nursing care of adults, children, and the child-bearing family; perioperative nursing; mental health nursing; community health nursing; nursing management and leadership; nursing theory; nursing research; nursing history and philosophy; and professional nursing concepts, issues, and development. As with ADN programs, critical thinking, ethical decision making, and problem solving are integrated into nursing courses.

Graduates of ADN and diploma programs may, as registered nurses, enter completion or mobility programs found within baccalaureate nursing programs. These types of programs build on the nursing experiences their students have, and students complete the educational requirements for the baccalaureate degree.

Graduates of all three nursing programs take the same licensure examination—the NCLEX-RN. Individuals passing this examination may use the initials R.N. after their name and are allowed to practice or work as a registered nurse in the state that issued the license. This is usually in the state in which the NCLEX-RN is successfully written. Registered nurses may hold multiple licenses to practice in multiple states.

Technicians Versus Generalists

Even though graduates of all three types of nursing programs write the same licensure examination, there is a difference in the focus of each program and in the overall abilities of the graduate. Associate degree and diploma programs prepare graduates for technical nursing practice. These graduates are viewed as care givers in structured care settings. The focus of their care is the individual patient or client.

Baccalaureate programs prepare graduates for professional nursing practice. These nurses are considered generalists because of their ability to perform diverse roles in various health care settings. Baccalaureate programs ask the most of their students, and society expects the most of its graduates. Baccalaureate graduates, in addition to being care givers, also serve as educators in vocational or practical nursing programs, researchers, case managers, client advocates, leaders, and consultants. Generalists deal with the individual patient or client, an individual family or group of families, groups of individuals, populations within communities, or entire communities. Generalists practice in both structured and unstructured health care settings.

Graduate Education

The baccalaureate degree in nursing is the stepping stone to graduate education. Many jobs require advanced education at the master's level and/or doctoral level.

Master's level programs prepare nurses for roles as educators in ADN, diploma, or baccalaureate nursing programs; researchers; managers or administrators in institutional or health care settings; or nurse practitioners. Master's programs in nursing are usually two years in length, providing the individual attends full time.

Doctoral programs offer professional degrees such as the Doctor of Education (Ed.D.), Doctor of Nursing Science (D.N.Sc.), and Doctor of Nursing (N.D.), and research degrees such as the Doctor of Philosophy (Ph.D.). Doctoral programs prepare master's educated nurses to practice as nurse educators in undergraduate and graduate nursing programs, administrators in health care or nonhealth care related settings, advanced clinical researchers, consultants, and independent practitioners.

Getting into Nursing School

Entry into a nursing program is dependent upon many factors—grade point average, SAT/ACT scores, references, interviews, writing ability, community or public service, and entrance examinations.

Admission is often competitive and schools of nursing may accept only those individuals who, according to the school's standardized criteria, have the greatest promise of success. Nursing schools typically have set standards for the number of admissions each academic year. For this reason, it is a good idea to apply to more than one school.

High school or community college grades are extremely important, and the higher the grade point average, the better. Many schools of nursing require a specific grade point average for consideration for entry into their programs. Most schools require a "B" or "C" average.

It is important to remember that having the required grade point average does not guarantee admission. For example, if the applicant pool for a particular academic year has an average grade point of 3.1 on a 4.0 scale, an individual with a grade point average of 2.0 who meets admission standards may not be granted admission. This is not because this individual could not succeed, but that other more qualified individuals were admitted.

ACT or SAT scores are utilized as admission criteria for many schools of nursing. Again, the higher your score, the better your chances of being admitted.

Most schools require a number of references. Your references should speak to your critical thinking and problem solving skills, your ability to master difficult and challenging content and material, and your ability to stick with and complete a project with or without difficult circumstances. You should be selective when asking for references and seek them from qualified, appropriate individuals, such as science or math teachers, professors, or better yet, from teachers whose honors or college prep courses you took. Employers may be good references if they are acquainted with your abilities to think logically, solve problems, and work responsibly.

Poor and inappropriate references are family, personal friends, and neighbors. The clergy may also be a poor source. These individuals know you personally and may be biased when it comes to your abilities.

Many schools of nursing require a personal interview as part of the admission process. If you go to one, make sure that you arrive 15 to 20 minutes early and look your best. Wear business-oriented clothing, not what is fashionable at the moment. Remove visible body piercings. Visible tattoos should be covered. Look and act professionally. Don't chew gum or suck on hard candy during your interview. Remember, the interviewers not only will be listening to what you have to say and how you say it but also will be critiquing how you look and present yourself.

A handwritten essay on a selected topic may be required. Reviewers are interested in your writing and reasoning abilities as well as your proficiency to discuss on paper a topic either known or unknown to you.

Some schools of nursing may be interested in the types of public or community service you've done. Performance of such service demonstrates an interest in society as a whole and indicates a well-rounded individual.

Nursing school entrance examinations may be required for admission to a school or such examinations may be taken afterward to provide further specific information. In either case, advance preparation is essential for high test scores.

If a school of nursing requires a nursing entrance examination as a part of or after the admission process, it will supply the necessary information and registration forms.

Special Testing Considerations

It is imperative that at this point in preparing for entrance into a nursing program, you identify early whether a learning disability exists, so that assistance is provided that will assist in your success with this examination, as well as those who are to follow once accepted into a program. For example, if you deal with extreme episodes of test anxiety during any testing, you will want to acknowledge this and get assistance that will help with the problem. Experiencing some test anxiety is expected and will provide alertness in making appropriate decisions; however, greater than this is extreme anxiety that may interfere with your thinking process to the point of difficulty focusing and concentrating. There are techniques that can assist in this situation. Your program will be able to guide you and make appropriate referrals that will assist toward success once you provide such information to them.

There are some students who will not help themselves by communicating their learning disability to the professors because of fear that friends will use such information against them or make them feel like they don't fit in or are "not smart." This is untrue. I have not experienced this with any of my numerous students who were helped as a result of sharing their learning disability with me. All students who identified their learning disabilities were provided assistance and have gone on to be successful in nursing.

If you have been diagnosed with a learning disability and have appropriate documentation supporting this fact, along with notification to the board of nursing, you will be offered special testing accommodations. In addition to board of nursing approval, the National Council of State Boards of Nursing (NCSBN) reviews the documents as well for approval. This means that you will be afforded assistance during your NCLEX.

Financial Assistance

Cost is an important factor when considering a school of nursing. Baccalaureate programs, by their very nature, will be more expensive than diploma or ADN programs because of the length of time required to complete course work.

The decision to work or not while attending school is an important one. Nursing education at any level is expensive. Many students have to work in order to pay for their education. Ideally, a student who does not have to work can devote all of the time necessary for study, preparation, class attendance, and clinical experiences.

The majority of individuals coming into a nursing program do not realize the time and effort required to do well. Nursing students typically spend many more hours in daily study and preparation for classes and clinicals than do students in nonhealth-related disciplines. Clinicals may be scheduled for 6 to 12 hours a day for two to three days a week. Students who work 10+ hours a week rarely have adequate time to prepare the required work or care for themselves.

The ideal situation is not to work unless there is no other option available to cover the cost of your education. If you must work, try to get a job in the health care field.

> ### CONSIDER ALL COSTS
> When considering the cost of a nursing education, allow for the following expenses each semester or quarter:
>
> 1. Tuition and fees
> 2. Room and board, if any, including money for meals at clinical sites
> 3. Books and other supplementary materials. Nursing books are expensive and should be kept, not sold, because they serve as reference material for subsequent courses. A computer may also be required
> 4. Uniforms, lab coat, and shoes
> 5. Malpractice insurance, purchased through the school of nursing
> 6. Stethoscope, bandage scissors, a watch with a second hand, and other required equipment. Some items are bought only once and others need to be replaced periodically
> 7. Transportation and/or vehicle upkeep costs
> 8. Personal health screening
> 9. Miscellaneous, hidden, or unexpected expenses
> 10. Money for entertainment, recreation, and relaxation. All study and no fun can lead to burnout and failure

Whatever the cost of a nursing education, financial assistance is available in many forms and in various amounts. The institution or the school of nursing you attend can provide specific information.

Prior to accepting any financial assistance, make sure you understand the terms of the contract. Educational loans typically have low interest rates and must be repaid after graduation. Failure to repay can negatively affect your credit rating and may, at some point in time, result in forfeiture of your nursing license. Although this issue is currently being debated, keep in mind that you cannot practice as a nurse without a valid license.

Scholarships and grants may be available that do not require repayment. These sources may not be based upon financial need but may be intended for individuals with certain interests or other needs. Numerous scholarships and grants are provided by private individuals or groups, nursing associations, and the business sector.

Continued financial assistance is often contingent upon grade point average and number of credit hours taken each semester. Grade point averages falling below stated levels or failure to take or complete the required number of credit hours may cancel financial assistance, or require repayment.

CHAPTER 2

Test-Taking Strategies and Reasoning

To succeed at test taking, the proper frame of mind is essential. The repetitive practice drills offered here will build confidence and skill. Through practice, you will learn to rely on your strengths and to lessen the impact of your weaknesses. Confidence will also help you focus on the task at hand.

This chapter focuses on how to master test items on any topic. Therefore, the test items are not necessarily directly related to the topics covered on nursing school entrance examinations but are instead intended to give you practice with various techniques for choosing correct responses on almost any topic.

The chapters that follow will give you more directed practice in the major topics that appear on nursing school entrance exams. When using this book, keep in mind that nursing school entrance exams vary in which major topics are covered. Your prospective nursing school will have selected which particular test, of the many available, meets its needs. So do not be dismayed if you studied all topics within this book and there were, say, no science questions on the particular nursing school entrance exam that you took. Practicing the sections of this book will help you to read carefully, sharpen your vocabulary, employ critical thinking skills, and complete test items in a timed way in preparation for whatever might appear on the actual entrance exam you will take.

This chapter will emphasize useful techniques for answering multiple-choice questions. It will assist you in learning to identify cues contained within questions. It will help you identify the three levels of knowledge called for within multiple-choice tests. You will practice techniques that will allow you to focus on essentials as you prepare to choose correctly from among responses. As you practice test-taking strategies, you will build your confidence in relying on the knowledge that you already have.

This chapter also highlights useful personal habits. An invaluable skill at test time is the ability to concentrate despite distractions and discomfort. Because of the need to maintain your focus at test time, you develop effective personal habits and mental strategies designed to fit your own personality during the weeks prior to testing.

At the end of this chapter, there is a very short and informal diagnostic test designed to identify areas requiring review. Though you may discover areas in which your recall from past educational activities is strong, there may be other areas in which you will need to review. The short diagnostic test is also intended to motivate you to refresh your memory about basic terms and other points of knowledge.

Before studying specific areas of knowledge, we will begin with some test-taking strategies for recognizing what any test question is asking. This will involve identifying levels of knowledge called for by the test item, employing critical thinking strategies, and then formulating a response.

Mastering Test Items

When a nurse must make a decision, a technique called critical thinking is often employed. A modification of this technique is used in this book. Critical thinking involves careful consideration of several available choices in order to select the best alternative. For example, if a test item asks what a nurse should deal with *first*, the reader is being asked to prioritize. If given two "patient discomfort" choices—a life-threatening situation such as a patient gasping for air, or a situation involving an angry family member—the well-educated nurse will first deal with the response that represents a life-threatening emergency: the patient with air hunger. One arrives at this choice through the careful and deliberative process known as critical thinking.

Critical thinking is based, usually, on the latest scientific knowledge combined with the use of logic skills. Using current knowledge in this way is termed *evidence-based practice*. As each test item within this book is tried and mastered, you will develop skill at critical thinking through use of logic and acquisition of the knowledge provided.

Beyond knowledge base and logic skills in such things as prioritization, there are additional strategies that will help the test taker to puzzle through difficult test items. These strategies involve careful reading of the stem of the question, paying attention to qualifying words within the stem, avoiding responses with extremes in language such as "always" and "never," and relying on first choices.

Careful rereading of the stem of the question is necessary when one is unable to easily select a correct response. Whether the stem is one sentence or a lengthy paragraph, slowly and carefully read each word once more. To provide clarifying details, it may even be helpful to visualize the "scene" with a particularly complex question. For example, with a health question, one might try to visualize a clinic or hospital room and an actual patient and visitors.

It is also helpful to pay close attention to any qualifying words such as "first" or "most" or "usually." Particularly with difficult test questions, these words can help the reader to lean toward a probable correct response or to avoid an incorrect response.

The reader should try to avoid responses with extreme wording such as "always" or "never." In the scientific community cautious language such as "usually" or "in most cases" is more frequently used. Therefore, correct responses on tests are often phrased with this more cautious language. Another extreme to avoid is assigning cause and effect. To say that one thing causes another can be a mistake. To say that two things are associated is more in keeping with scientific thought. So beware of absolutes when deciding on a response.

Finally, some test-taking authorities recommend staying with the first answer chosen. In other words, select a response and do not rethink the choice too much. Do not change an answer once it is selected. The thought is that the brain's hemispheres work in concert at the moment a decision is made. This affords the test taker a unique moment of selecting the correct choice.

Levels of Test Questions

The first strategy for improving multiple-choice test scores involves recognition of what the test question, also called the test item, is asking. With current, nationally standardized, multiple-choice tests, you are asked to examine a test item and then select one answer from among four possible responses provided. There are always four possible responses. By narrowing choices down to fewer than the four provided, you can focus on the ones that are most likely to be correct. If you can narrow your choices down to two from among the four provided, your chances of selecting the best response, even if you knew nothing about the subject matter, would improve dramatically. Techniques for narrowing and eliminating will be highlighted later in this chapter.

Another useful strategy is understanding the levels of test items used with multiple-choice tests. The three levels are recall, application, and analysis. Being able to recognize the level allows you to concentrate on the method you will use to answer the question.

The Recall Level of Test Question

Recall level, considered the least complex, involves remembering a piece of information. It does not ask you to do anything with the information; it asks only that you recall something from the set of facts you bring to the test.

For example:

1. Which of the following is the best definition of *trauma*?

    (A) Illness
    (B) A disease or disorder requiring health care
    (C) Injury
    (D) Mishap; unfortunate occurrence

The response to this question is fairly straightforward. You simply need to know that trauma relates to injury rather than an illness (choice A) or disease (choice B). Once you have eliminated the two poor choices, you are left with only two other possibilities. After a little more thought, you will probably select choice C because it implies that there was damage done, rather than just a negative occurrence (choice D).

When you recognize an item as a recall question, you can either respond immediately, if you have the knowledge, or go on to the narrowing phase. The narrowing process is described in more detail shortly. Recall-level test items are easily recognizable. Either you know it or you don't.

MEMORY AIDS IN INFORMATION RECALL

What if you were asked to respond to a recall-level test item involving the term *degeneration*? If you have instant recall of the information, then your task is simple. You select the definition from among the choices provided.

For example:

2. The term *degeneration* relates to which of the following?

   (A) Negentropy
   (B) Building up, multiplying
   (C) Hair loss
   (D) Decomposition

The correct response to this recall-level question would be decomposition, choice D. The item was probably simple for you. But what if you cannot recall what degeneration means? You have two choices. One is to move on to the next item. Sometimes this is wise if you are taking the type of paper-and-pencil test that allows you to return to a particular item. However, some computerized tests do not allow you to skip an item without penalty. And some may not allow you to return to a skipped item. So, time permitting, another option is to use a memory trick recommended by some psychologists. Simply concentrate on something else for just a few seconds. When you return your attention to the subject at hand, the lost piece of information may suddenly pop into your mind. This is similar to the situation in which you lose your car keys, do something else, and then remember where they are.

However, this particular memory trick is not always useful. Some types of information take longer for recall, such as names of prior acquaintances, certain diseases, or names of celebrities that are right "on the tip of your tongue." Unfortunately, these tend to pop into your mind several days later, if at all. So, do not continue using this trick if the information does not return fairly easily and quickly. And do not be dismayed when the lost information comes to mind later on in the test. Realize that this is just the way the mind works. Console yourself with the thought that, possibly, other test takers are having the same problem.

TIP

Sometimes the difference between good recall and not being able to remember relates to good personal habits leading up to the test. Cramming, loss of sleep, or poor diet may actually hinder your ability to remember.

NARROWING AND ELIMINATING

Another technique called the narrowing strategy can be used in the case of the lost-to-memory test item. In order to understand how this works, you first have to understand the reasoning behind the multiple-choice selections. From among the four choices provided, you can expect to see: one correct response, two obviously incorrect responses, and one distractor. The two incorrect responses are there to ensure that you have some knowledge of the subject being tested. If you select one of these, you didn't have a starting point, or a clue, for responding. The distractor item is something that is close to correct, but not quite. It is there to ensure that your understanding of the topic has a bit of depth. In the case of our example dealing with *degeneration*, you might recall that the term has something to do with breaking down, or rotting. As such, you can eliminate choice B, building up. You may also eliminate choice A since you either are not sure what it means, or you recall that it involves the creation of order from disorder, which would be the opposite of degeneration. By narrowing your choices to two, you have increased your chances of being correct.

Practice with Recall Questions

Directions: Choose the best answer.

1. Upon hearing that you might become a nurse, an 84-year-old person, who lives with his daughter and her family, asks you whether giving up smoking would be a good idea at such an advanced age. Which of the following would be a response most likely to encourage this particular person to stop smoking?

   (A) Cigarettes cost a lot of money.
   (B) It has been found that second-hand smoke may be associated with illness in those who are near to the smoker.
   (C) It probably doesn't matter once a person turns 60 or so.
   (D) There are tremendous health benefits when you give up smoking at any age.

2. Which of the following is accurate about the boiling point of water? Water boils at:

   (A) 100 degrees Fahrenheit.
   (B) 0 degrees Fahrenheit.
   (C) 100 degrees Centigrade.
   (D) Minus 217 degrees Fahrenheit.

3. Risk factors closely identified with the development of cardiovascular disease include which of the following?

   (A) Eating spicy foods
   (B) Air pollution
   (C) Frequent childhood illnesses, such as measles and colds
   (D) Family history of heart disease

4. A leading cause of death among teenagers in the United States is:

   (A) amyotrophic lateral sclerosis.
   (B) cancer.
   (C) cardiovascular disease.
   (D) accidents.

Answers:

1. **(B)** You can rule out choice C, that it just does not matter, since the aim is to encourage the person to give up smoking. Now you can devote your attention to the remaining choices.

Choice A, concerning money saved, may or may not appeal to this individual, depending on his financial situation. So it is safe to eliminate this response.

It is likely that choice B would appeal to the individual's sense of doing something good for the family. Choice D, health benefits, is uncertain. Giving up smoking might have no effect, or given his age, the individual may not care to go through the process of smoking cessation.

By eliminating alternatives, you are more likely to select the appropriate response.

2. **(C)** In this example, you may know the correct temperature. However, even if you did not, you could arrive at the correct choice through process of elimination, or visualization. Pretend you're looking at a thermometer and reading possible temperatures in winter and summer. Since freezing is 32 degrees Fahrenheit or zero degrees Celsius, you can rule out choices B and D. Both are colder than the freezing point and, therefore, would not cause water to boil.

This leaves choices A and C. Once again, picture a thermometer on a hot summer day. It might be as warm as 100 degrees Fahrenheit, but it is not hot enough to cause water to boil. This rules out choice A. Therefore, only choice C (100 degrees Centigrade) remains.

3. **(D)** Again, try to rule out obviously incorrect responses and visualize yourself in the situation. Since no one falls to the ground in the throes of heart disease just from eating spicy food, you can rule out choice A.

Choice B seems possible. Air pollution has been known to cause health problems. So this response cannot be ruled out yet.

Choice C might bring to mind children with communicable diseases, perhaps at the turn of the century, lying in large hospital wards. But does everyone who has had mumps or head colds go on to develop heart disease? No.

Now you're left with two reasonable choices: B and D. In considering choice D, picture a scenario in which both sets of grandparents died in old age of heart or vascular diseases and in which your mother states that no diabetes, cancer, or other illnesses run in the family. What will you conclude? The answer is fairly straightforward. Family history has been linked to development of heart disease in the individual.

4. **(D)** You may simply recall that accidents (choice D) are the leading cause of death among teenagers in the United States. But suppose you do not know that. Narrowing and elimination will help. Choices A and B may both be eliminated. Choice A is not frequently mentioned, and choice B usually applies to people over the age of 45.

By eliminating these two choices, the chance of a correct response is 50% (50–50), even without any knowledge of whether heart disease or accidents are the leading cause of death in teenagers. To pinpoint the correct response, recall your high school years. How did one of your classmates die? Chances are that person was killed in an automobile accident. This leads to the correct answer—accidents.

The Application Level of Test Question

The second and more difficult level of test item is application. Here, you are asked to do something with the knowledge you have. Typically, you are asked what you would do in a real situation. For example, you might be asked to select the best way to save yourself in case of a shipwreck. Based on your knowledge of survival, you would choose from a list of four possible responses.

For example:

1. You are about to be shipwrecked and have a chance to select the three most important items to take to a nearby desert island. You know that coconuts, bananas, mammalian creatures, and water are present there. Which would be most important for survival?

   (A) A book on how to cook foods from scratch, a sharp knife, and string
   (B) A gun, mosquito netting, and a compass
   (C) A flare gun with a supply of six flares, matches, and a sharp knife
   (D) String, sharp knife, and matches

Choice D is correct. Since the test item never mentions bullets for the gun, and the cookbook is optional, you can rule out choices A and B. Choices C and D remain attractive, but, with a bit of thought, you realize you're not going to kill island beasts with a knife. That leaves fish as a source of protein, which you might be able to catch with string.

Another application-level item would ask you to read a short paragraph and then ask you what you would do.

Practice with Application Questions

Directions: Read the passage and then choose the best answer.

1. You have arrived recently in a tropical city as a student. You are on a scholarship and have barely enough money to make ends meet. You must work part-time while going to school and have very little time to study or to commute.

   This is a city of contrasts. Each day, you must drive to your school, through stressful traffic and amidst loudly honking horns, but around lovely parks and monuments. Although there are signs of wealth everywhere, you also find yourself in the midst of street people who rap on your windows and beg for money. This is a prosperous Western world city, yet these are some of its more unfortunate citizens. You feel uneasy about giving money because it could be used to purchase illicit substances. You have heard that there is a large substance abuse problem in this city. Or perhaps, if you give the money, you might feel that you were coerced. There is a genuine sense of unease.

Which of the following alternatives makes the most sense in this situation?

(A) Give the money with the thought that, perhaps in some cases, it will do some good. You argue that you can afford nickels and dimes.
(B) Give the money because you feel intimidated. These people might get angry if you don't give them something.
(C) Instead of money, give sandwiches that you've carefully prepared each morning.
(D) Give nothing, frown, and blow the horn loudly when people approach.

Answer:

The set-up paragraph gives clues to the most sensible response. You know that you have no extra money and no time. Therefore, choices A, B, and C, involving giving money or sandwiches, will not work. Although you're not in total accord with the remaining alternative, involving blowing your horn and warning people off, you feel that it's perhaps the only solution among the choices given.

In your classes at the tropical city's university, you learn that, in making choices involving moral principles, there are guidelines. Some of these involve principles such as beneficence, justice, and respect for autonomy. You know that you have an oversimplified grasp of these principles but decide to try to place your recent choice in context. Which of the following would most closely fit the method you have just chosen, that of honking and keeping people away?

(A) Beneficence, or doing good works
(B) Justice, which could be said to equate to fairness and a "level playing field for all"
(C) Autonomy, or free will: the right to do as one wants, contingent on not infringing on the rights of others
(D) Separation of church and state

Choice C is correct. Even with a minimal knowledge of ethical principles, the test taker will recognize that the other responses do not apply to the method chosen.

Application questions such as these involve two steps. The first is deciding what you know about the general topic. The second is selecting an action from the various possibilities offered. With practice at recognizing application questions, you will be able to sort through what you know about the category and then consider which response fits your store of knowledge.

The Analysis Level of Test Question

The third level of difficulty is called analysis. You are typically asked to break a situation down into its component parts, examine their interactions, and then select the best response from the four offered. Analysis is considered complex.

To analyze effectively, you need to read the test item and then decide what information is needed.

For example:

1. You are driving an automobile and see what could be a tornado on the far horizon. What is the most important priority at this moment?

    (A) Drive in the direction of the possible tornado to confirm that what you are seeing is, in fact, a tornado.
    (B) Get out of your car and lie down in a nearby ditch.
    (C) Find a highway overpass and, abandoning your car, seek shelter underneath.
    (D) Drive away from the possible tornado, generally at right angles to the direction in which the tornado is moving.

In responding to this question, you need to have at least three different types of information at your disposal. You should know the dynamics of tornadoes. How do they move? At what rate do they travel? Do they change direction with extreme rapidity? In other words, will you have time to change your mind should the strategy you choose not work?

Next, you should know what the best type of protection is in case the tornado catches up with you—ditch, underpass, or car? You should also know whether a car can outrun a tornado.

First, decide whether all four responses are worth considering. After you examine each response, you decide that you cannot rule any out. Your first analysis step is complete. You compared choices with your current store of knowledge about tornadoes and decided that any of the choices could be correct so you need to continue to consider all four.

You decide to analyze the next simplest type of information. What do you know about tornadoes and what would make you feel most comfortable in this situation? Or, an even more fine-tuned type of analysis would lead you to ask who else would be answering this question and what kind of information would they have on hand. What would high schools all over the country and television shows be teaching about tornadoes? What do real people do to decide in such an emergency? You try to place yourself in the situation. You decide that, since the tornado is on the horizon (meaning far away at the moment), your best chance and the thing that makes you feel most comfortable is to drive away from it. This actually is the best answer. Hiding may be something you have to do later. You know that, should the tornado overtake you, a car is no match and you may have to duck under that overpass or find a ditch. But, for now, running away feels pretty good. The idea of driving in the direction of the tornado never felt right. So you correctly select choice D.

Your task, when confronted with an analysis-level test item, usually falls into two parts. First decide what realms of knowledge the question is asking you to dredge forth. Examine each in turn, looking for a clue to a correct response. If you can rule anything out, then do so immediately and concentrate on the others.

After you have examined each response, then perform the second part. Take what you think has the highest chance of being correct, based on your knowledge, and what you think is the typical knowledge level of all others taking the same test and respond. Analysis-level questions are considered to be the most difficult types to answer. If you feel unsure of your answer, you can be certain that other test takers feel the same. Sometimes, as with the tornado item, you place yourself in a given situation and go with your gut. In other words, select what would feel right to you in a real situation.

A brief section of practice items follows. Additional opportunities for practice with analysis-level test items are provided in subsequent chapters. As you practice analysis-type responses, remember that you are similar to the athlete in training who visualizes a ball being hit or being speedy at take-off. Not only are you trying to understand the basis of each test item, but you are developing a sense of automaticity, or what swimming teachers call muscle memory. After much practice, beginning swimmers learn to stroke and breathe and kick automatically. The same happens with test taking. Although practice with test items seems tedious, if you practice, you will be able to break down questions more quickly, and your confidence will build. As in the real world of nursing decision making, both knowledge and timing are important. To develop your ability to sustain your mental energy for the duration of a test, practice is important. We urge you to rely on subsequent chapters for drill and practice that will produce test-taking success.

Practice with Analysis Questions

Directions: Read the paragraphs that follow and select the best answers to individual questions, based on information in the paragraphs.

A banker must make a decision about how much an individual buyer will be allowed to borrow in order to purchase a house. We'll term this a long-term loan, or long-term debt.

A common way that bankers determine how much long-term debt an individual can safely assume involves calculating the percentage of after-tax income the individual makes each month. The banker then uses a rule involving percentages.

The first of three ways in which relative purchasing power might be determined involves calculating 15 to 20 percent of after-tax monthly income. This percentage, which we will term medium-term debt, should be the ceiling for all monthly loan-related expenditures, exclusive of mortgage payments. In other words, with medium-term debt, the homeowner should be paying no more than 20 percent of monthly income on such things as car payments, credit debt, or other types of loans. Bankers try to rule out giving a loan to anyone who is overextended financially. No one who pays more than 20 percent of income on medium-term debts will find it easy to obtain a mortgage.

The second method of figuring long-term debt allowances involves calculating 33 to 36 percent of monthly after-tax income. In performing this maneuver, bankers count the monthly mortgage payment and all other debt (long-term and medium-term) as they calculate how much expense is possible for the house payment. In this case, all monthly debt payments, including the monthly house payment (principal, interest, taxes, and insurance, or PITI) are calculated. If the resulting number does not exceed 36 percent of after-tax income, the house is usually considered affordable.

Finally, bankers check just the amount of the house payment. House payments should never exceed 25 to 28 percent of monthly income.

1. Audra and Mac have been spending Sundays looking at houses. They both work. Audra makes $2000 a month after taxes and Mac brings home $1500. They have worked at their jobs for 11 years and are considered a stable couple. They just found a house they like, and the realtor tells them that PITI will amount to $750, provided that they come up with a pre-agreed down payment. Using the rule of 25 to 28 percent, will the banker be likely to loan them the money?

   (A) Yes. Their monthly payment is affordable.
   (B) No. Their monthly payment would be too high.
   (C) It can't be determined without knowing the size of the down payment.
   (D) None of the above.

2. The banker next looks at their total monthly debt to determine if the loan is safe. This couple owns one car and makes payments of $199 per month on a second car, which will be paid off in three years. They have a $250 balance on a department store credit card and pay the minimum of $10 per month. The approximate percentage of monthly debt, not counting the mortgage (PITI) will be:

   (A) 23 percent.
   (B) 18 percent.
   (C) 2 percent.
   (D) 6 percent.

3. Finally, the banker examines the percentage of all monthly debt. What will be the outcome?

   (A) The bank will make the loan since total debt is 15 percent of monthly income.
   (B) The bank will make the loan since total debt is 27 percent of monthly income.
   (C) The bank will not make the loan since total debt is 40 percent of monthly income.
   (D) The bank will make the loan since total debt is 40 percent of monthly income.

4. Which of the following is logical in relation to why firehouses have circular stairways?

   (A) Firemen can slide down.
   (B) Horses, in the old days, couldn't climb up.
   (C) Firehouses don't have circular staircases.
   (D) Stairways were made out of metal to prevent combustion and because the weight of the traditional style of stairway would have been prohibitive.

Answers:

1. **(A)** Audra and Mac can afford their dream house. Let's review why the banker will approve their loan.

    Recall that analysis questions ask you to focus on your knowledge concerning the matter at hand. You need to set aside the extraneous information and examine the 25 to 28 percent rule. By calculating 28 percent of their $3500 income (multiplying 0.28 by $3500), you know that Audra and Mac can afford a house with up to $980 in monthly payments. Because the $750 mortgage payment falls below this ceiling, you can be sure that a banker would be likely to approve the loan.

    Even if you feel overwhelmed by a problem that seems too complex, you can place yourself in the situation. For example, you can picture yourself standing in front of a pay window and watching someone count out thirty-five $100 bills. That is the exact amount that Audra and Mac earn. Next, you can visualize yourself driving up to the bank's mortgage window and surrendering $800 to make a house payment of $750. After you get your $50 in change, will you still have three quarters of your money left?

    To answer this question, you must picture four piles of money with a little less than $900 in each pile so that the four piles total $3500. You would need to keep three fourths of that money in order to afford the mortgage. You know that parting with just under $800 for your mortgage means that you will keep at least three piles, or 75 percent of your money. Using the visualization method, you can also conclude that Audra and Mac will soon be moving into their new home.

2. **(D)** Again, you are asked to sift through the introductory paragraphs and assemble information related to the question. This time you need to underline or highlight the information concerning total monthly debt. Because you are told not to include mortgage in this total, you add the car payment and the $10 credit card payment (not the balance) and come up with $209 in monthly expenses. To find out what percentage of monthly income this is, divide the $209 by $3500, which is 6 percent or choice D.

    You may want to double-check yourself using the visualization method. First, picture the 20 percent limit on medium-term debt. You will have to calculate it by multiplying 0.20 by $3500. You should determine that Audra and Mac could be spending as much as $700 on medium-term debt and still qualify for the home loan. Or you can picture yourself counting out $3500 into five piles of money (each is one fifth or 20 percent of monthly income). You wind up putting $700 in each pile. So again you know that Audra and Mac can afford the roughly $200 in debt.

    Visualizing the problem may seem like a silly and unnecessary step, but using it can prevent you from making an obvious mistake. Nursing students are often taught this technique to double check themselves when they are calculating dosages, solutions, or IV running rates. It is a good habit to get into.

3. **(B)** Total debt is only 27 percent of monthly income; the house is affordable. You know from your reading that up to 36 percent could be spent on all debt.

To calculate total debt, you need to add up all projected debt ($209 plus $750, or $959) and then divide $959 by $3500. This gives you the 27 percent figure.

To visualize and check yourself, you picture 36 percent of all your money (about one third) lying in piles on the floor. You have three piles of money, with each pile containing one third of your money, or about $1200. You need to spend no more than one of these piles on all debt. So you add up all your projected debt to see if it wipes out any more than one $1200 pile. Eureka! The $959 of debt payment means you'll have some money left over each month.

4. **(B)** Considering each response in turn, your recall that firefighters traditionally slide down poles, not staircases. That eliminates choice A. You picture the old days of firehouses and recall horses drawing red metal firewagons. So you do not rule this choice out yet. You do not like choices C and D. The first is untrue, and the second one seems too complicated and also is probably untrue. Going back to choice B, you decide that horses were probably stabled on the first floor of the firehouse and that, if a stairway was straight, the hungry or companionable horses would eventually figure out that they could climb the stairs and join the humans.

Summary

Our discussion of levels of test questions has involved somewhat easy and tongue-in-cheek examples, but the actual test will involve more complicated thinking in a less congenial atmosphere. If you practice with the sample test items at the back of this book, you will develop solid test-taking skill and will be able to relax in the face of complex questions. When you find yourself confused by a question you will have experience using the visualization method. You will be able to picture yourself in the situation with all the items that you need to have to look for the parts of the question that are important. Finally, you will be well rested and in good health. The next section addresses that most important area.

Developing Effective Personal Habits to Enhance Test Skills

In addition to preparing that store of knowledge you have built up through the years for a major test situation, you must put yourself into the best condition for retrieving thoughts and using logic skills. If you know quite a bit but are unable to summon it when needed, through either a lack of concentration or a type of mental blocking, then it becomes difficult to succeed.

Conditioning Yourself Before the Test

In order to maximize your chances of successful concentration and skilled retrieval of information or effective use of logic skills at the time of testing, you should be in peak physical and mental condition. You should also be able to minimize negative emotional factors that might cause a loss of confidence or of concentration at test time. It is natural to be jittery before the exam, but overwhelming fatigue or anxiety can cause a definite but avoidable decline in performance.

The body-brain complex prefers plenty of sleep and a nutritious diet. So, if you know that you are within ten days of a test situation, it is worth your time and effort to ensure that your favorite nutritious foods and perhaps some multiple vitamins are available so that the study and stress do not take too much of a toll on you. In addition, although the idea of staying up for all-nighters may seem compelling, the lack of sleep usually drops your concentration and comfort at test time. Things that are normally easily recalled or logic that is soundly used under normal circumstances fall away, as you sit uncomfortably, unable to concentrate sufficiently during the test.

In addition to a good night's sleep in each of the days leading up to test time, you may need to use "both sides" of the brain when studying. Have you noticed that, when immersed in logic and memorization, the mind tends to want to drift? If you have been studying for hours and have not relaxed your mind, you may be fighting human nature. You may want to set a clock or timer to periodically signal the start of a relaxation period and, later, to recall you to the task at hand after you have allowed yourself to drift or daydream or play a computer game or listen to uplifting music. Indeed, some people can listen to music while they use logic and memorization skills in intensive study. So do not begrudge yourself periodic breaks or simultaneous exposure to things that stimulate the creative and pleasure-seeking areas of your mind.

As you are studying, you should also "feed" the mind to ensure alertness. It is often useful to have quickly absorbed nutrients on hand as you study. Because fats and proteins may take longer to be absorbed, carbohydrates are useful. When you are studying, the mind uses nutrients and oxygen more purposefully, so ensuring good supplies of both is advisable.

Getting Started on the Day of the Test

We consider the night before the test as part of the immediate period surrounding the testing situation. So, in order to ensure relaxation, a positive spirit, and a good night's sleep, the usual rules apply. *Stop studying.* It is in your best interest to sleep soundly before a test, so try to do something relaxing, beginning after dinner, the day before the exam. You may also want to use dairy products liberally. A substance contained in these products is known to enhance your ability to sleep. To allay nervousness, tell yourself that there will be many other test takers, against whom you are being measured, who are far less prepared than you are. Finally, if you cannot sleep, try to find something to read for pleasure, not for studying purposes. It will help to clear away some of the cobwebs and may help you fall asleep.

On the big day, start early, make sure your nutrition levels are up, and arrive early at the test site.

Following these test preparation methods will enhance your ability to concentrate and to succeed at achieving the highest possible score on the day of the test. Because there is no substitute for knowledge of the subjects upon which you will be tested, the following chapters offer you a chance to practice identifying types of test items and narrowing response possibilities. Subsequent chapters will direct your efforts at studying certain topics. There will be suggestions for scoring yourself and for determining what you should be studying. Although nothing can guarantee absolute success, practice with the book will enhance the abilities you already have.

Short Diagnostic Test

This section is designed to alert you to any weaknesses in the major subject areas used in most nursing school entrance examinations. These test items will help you to recall terms and basic knowledge from the four major nursing school entrance exam subject areas: verbal, mathematics, science, and reading comprehension. Although there is no formal score for this short diagnostic test, if you are unable to recall how to answer an item or if you respond incorrectly, you will want to review that area of knowledge. And, although it is recommended that you use the entire book for review, you may want to begin your studies with subject areas in which you identified potential weaknesses.

I. VERBAL ABILITY

1. Identify the word that is spelled correctly from the list.

   (A) regretable
   (B) regretible
   (C) regrettable
   (D) regrettible

2. Identify the pair of synonyms.

   (A) muddy - lucid
   (B) opaque - reflective
   (C) reticent - flashy
   (D) ephemeral - fleeting

II. MATH

1. Add the following numbers: 5,482 plus 28 plus 64,873

2. Solve for X: 75 mg: 50 ml = 225 mg: X ml

3. What is the area of the rectangle if the four sides are 8 feet, 3 feet, 8 feet, and 3 feet in length?

III. SCIENCE

1. Identify the terms that are examples of genus and species nomenclature.

   (A) primus arachnis
   (B) Bella Fortuna
   (C) Kingdom and phylum
   (D) Mycobacterium tuberculae

2. Neutral pH is:
   (A) 4.0
   (B) 3.5 to 4.5
   (C) 7.0
   (D) 8.5

IV. READING COMPREHENSION

A classification of respiratory disorders is known as restrictive. Although there are a variety of specific disorders that fall into this classification, they all have one thing in common. Disease or injury has overcome the usual propensity of the chest to return, passively (without expenditure of energy), to a relaxed position at the end of expiration. From the list provided, identify the disorders that would be classified as restrictive respiratory disorders. There may be more than one within the listing.

(A) upper respiratory infection
(B) black lung (miner's lung) disease
(C) fractured ribs
(D) all of the above

Answers:

I. VERBAL ABILITY

1. **(C)**
2. **(D)**

II. MATH

1. 70,383
2. 150
3. 24 square feet

III. SCIENCE

1. **(D)**
2. **(C)**

IV. READING COMPREHENSION

Responses B and C are the most likely. A case could be made that any infection causes discomfort with exhalation, but the others in the list are more likely to result in much energy expenditure to complete the act of breathing out. Incidentally, this test item involved the reader's ability to infer a response from the brief information in the paragraph combined with common knowledge of diseases.

Verbal Ability

One of the most important skills that a registered nurse can have is the ability to communicate effectively with patients, families, and other health care workers. Verbal ability, or the capacity to use and comprehend spoken language competently, forms the basis of effective communication and is necessary for success in everyday life.

Communication based on weak verbal ability places all involved at risk. For example, someone may misunderstand what was said and feel offended. A nurse may misinterpret a physician's verbal order and give a patient an incorrect treatment. Effective communication may cease between nurse and patient or between nurse and other health care workers if the nurse cannot listen carefully and speak concisely.

Enhance What You Already Have

There are many techniques to increase your verbal ability. Start with increasing your vocabulary. Make this activity a part of your everyday learning and conversation.

There are a number of strategies that you might employ to increase your vocabulary:

1. Write new or undefinable words you hear or see in a notebook and look them up in a dictionary. Write out all the definitions because words frequently have a number of different meanings and can be used in many different ways. Consider the word *pass*:

    The highway sign said, "Do not *pass*."
    The quarterback threw a long *pass* to a receiver.
    The child asked his mother to *pass* the green beans.
    The teacher hoped all the students would *pass* the test.
    Everyone thought the man would *pass* away since his condition had worsened.
    The mountain *pass* contained many obstacles for the climbers.
    The student requested a library *pass*.

2. Practice using new words in conversations with others to incorporate them into your vocabulary. Merely knowing how to define words strengthens your vocabulary only slightly. You must actively use the words to strengthen your vocabulary.

3. Read different types of materials to expose yourself to new words. Most public libraries subscribe to numerous newspapers, magazines, and trade journals. Find time each week to read articles with information unfamiliar to you. Take a dictionary with you and define new words as you encounter them. Remember to use these words in your daily conversations. British and Canadian spelling of some words is different than some American spellings. If you are planning to take entrance examinations for American schools of nursing, make sure that you learn the American spelling of words.

4. Attend lectures and speeches to hear others speak. Most public speakers have excellent vocabularies. Again, write down the new words, define them, and use them in your daily conversations with others.

5. Review self-help books on verbal ability. Such information may be contained in books dealing with vocabulary, grammar, and spelling.

6. Engage in activities that require you to spell correctly and know the meanings of words. Practice working crossword puzzles or playing board games such as Scrabble.

7. After you've defined and incorporated new words into your active vocabulary, consult a thesaurus or synonym-antonym finder to learn antonyms and synonyms of the words.

Etymology

Simply defined, etymology is the study of the origin or formation of words. All the words used in our daily speech and writing have come from other sources. Our words are a hodge-podge of words or word pieces from languages and times all over the world. Some words have existed for so long that they are considered as old as time, whereas other words can be traced back to a specific era in world history.

Words are not merely historical. New words are constantly being formulated or altered as technology and society changes. In the 1920s, the word *gay* had to do with happiness and merriment. Today the word *gay* is closely aligned with homosexuality and represents a distinctive lifestyle.

Words are often formed by putting together what might be considered word pieces or groups of letters. These pieces are prefixes, roots, and suffixes. If you understand these pieces, you can break down a specific word into its individual pieces or parts in order to define the word.

Prefixes

A prefix is a word, syllable, or group of letters that comes before a root word and alters the meaning of the word. Many prefixes come from Old English, Greek, Latin, and French. Prefixes have comprehensive, commonplace meanings like with, through, among, and beyond.

Consider the use of the prefix *dis* and the root word *obedient*. The prefix *dis* means not or the opposite of. *Obedient* means dutiful or obeying. An obedient child is one who is dutiful or obeys, whereas a disobedient child is one who does not behave or does not do what he is supposed to do. Our language contains hundreds of prefixes. Many are in common use and some are rarely used.

When adding a prefix to a root word, the spelling of the word remains the same. Consider the following examples using the prefixes *peri*, *hemi*, *co*, and *ultra*:

EXAMPLE

peri + scope = periscope
hemi + sphere = hemisphere
co + exist = coexist
ultra + modern = ultramodern

A partial list of common prefixes is provided in Table 3.1. To learn more prefixes, consult a dictionary or other source containing prefixes.

Table 3.1
Common Prefixes

Prefix	Meaning	Example
a	not; without	The article described the man as *amoral*.
ab	away from	The couple would *abstain* from sex until they were married.
ad	toward; to	All children looked forward to the *adventure*.
ante	before	Our telephone was in the *anteroom*.
anti	against	The woman supported the *antidemocracy* movement.
be	by; near	The child sat *beside* her mother.
bene	good; well	The man was *benevolent*.
bi	two	Many older adults wear *bifocals*.
circum	around; about	The planets in our solar system have a *circumsolar* orbit.
co	with; together	The man and woman were *coanchors* on the evening news.
com	together	The recipe said to *combine* the dry ingredients.
contra	against	The couple went to their doctor to discuss methods of *contraception*.
counter	opposite	During the debate, the woman made a *counter-proposal*.
de	from; down; away	The guard instructed the group to *descend* the stairs and turn right.
equi	equal	The river is *equidistant* between the two cities.
ex	out of; former	A woman was *excommunicated* from the church when she divorced her husband.

Table 3.1
Common Prefixes

Prefix	Meaning	Example
extra	beyond	The man was sure he saw an *extraterrestrial* being.
infra	below; beneath	The *infrastructure* of the building was damaged in the earthquake.
inter	between	Group *interaction* was better than expected.
intra	within	*Intramural* sports were offered in public schools.
macro	large	The scientist said proteins are *macromolecular*.
mal	bad	The infant was *malformed*.
mega	large	Nuclear explosions in heavily populated areas would cause *megadeath*.
micro	small	A student used a *microscope* to examine the fly's wing.
mid	middle	The family decided on a *midday* picnic.
mini	small	Our *minivan* was too small for family needs.
mis	wrong	There were many *misspellings* in the paper.
multi	many	The SAT is a *multiple*-choice exam.
non	not	The country was *nonaligned* during the war.
ob	against	No one on the committee would *object* to the rule changes.
over	excessive	The owner *overcharged* for the computer repair.
peri	around	The pregnant woman was entering the *perinatal* period.
poly	many	*Polygamy* is against the law in the United States.
post	after; later	A *posttest* was administered at the end of the seminar.
pre	before	The couple enrolled in *premarital* counseling courses.
pro	supporting	The man lived in a *procommunist* country.
pseudo	false	The woman published her books using a *pseudonym*.
re	again	Smart students *review* their notes the night before the exam.
retro	backward	Pay raises are *retroactive*.
semi	half	The recipe called for *semisweet* chocolate.
socio	social; society	*Sociology* class met three times a week.
sub	under	The building contractor offered four *subcontracts*.

Table 3.1
Common Prefixes

Prefix	Meaning	Example
super	above	Farmers had a *superabundant* harvest.
supra	above	The football player sustained a *supraorbital* injury.
trans	across	His goal was to enter a *transcountry* race.
ultra	beyond	The man was known as an *ultraconservative* politician.
un	not	Many of the groups activities were considered *un-American*.
under	beneath	The migrants were *underpaid* for their work.
vice	in place of; next to in rank	The woman listed her occupation as *vice president* of the company
with	against; back	The family asked the doctor to *withhold* medical treatment.

Suffixes

Suffixes are the opposite of prefixes and are found at the end of a root word instead of at the beginning. Suffixes do one of two things. They may create a new word, as when adding the suffix *dom* to the word *free* to make a new word *freedom*.

Suffixes may alter the original word in some fashion but not change the meaning of the word. Consider the suffix *ed* and the root word *edit*. The suffix *ed* changes a word from the present tense to the past tense. *Edit* means to correct or change. An edited paper is one that has been corrected or changed. The editing of the paper took place in the past instead of the present. The suffix *ed* does not tell when the editing took place, only that it occurred.

A number of mechanical rules apply to adding suffixes to root words.

1. When the suffix begins with a vowel, double the final consonant of the root word before the suffix—provided that the root word has only one syllable or the accent is on the last syllable.

   brag + g + art = braggart
   rob + b + ery = robbery
   regret + t + ing = regretting
   profit + able = profitable

2. When the suffix *less*, *ness*, *ly*, or *en* is added to a root word, the spelling of the root word does not change.

   heart + less = heartless
   fond + ness = fondness
   late + ly = lately
   wood + en = wooden

Exceptions to this rule are when the root word ends in *y* and the *y* changes to an *i* before the suffixes *ness* and *ly*.

```
dingy + ness = dingi + ness = dinginess
swarthy + ness = swarthi + ness = swarthiness
```

3. When the suffix begins with a vowel, drop the final *e* in the root words ending in *e*.

```
write + ing = writ + ing = writing
deflate + ing = deflat + ing = deflating
desire + able = desir + able = desirable
```

4. When the suffix begins with a consonant, keep the final *e* of root words ending with *e*.

```
lone + some = lonesome
hope + less = hopeless
state + hood = statehood
```

Exceptions to this are rule are words such as *judgment*, *acknowledgment*, and *argument*.

5. When root words end in *y* preceded by a consonant, change the *y* to *i* before adding the suffix. This applies to suffixes not starting with *i*.

```
beauty + ful = beauti + ful = beautiful
lazy + ness = lazi + ness = laziness
```

A partial list of common suffixes is found in Table 3.2. Consult a dictionary or other appropriate source for more suffixes.

Table 3.2
Common Suffixes

Suffix	Meaning	Example
ability	inclination for	The first lesson he learned at the academy was *respectability*.
able	worthy of an act	The woman was a *capable* leader.
ac	pertaining to	A *cardiac* muscle had ruptured.
acy	having the quality of	The team's target practice had an *accuracy* rate of 90 percent.
age	collection, connection	The museum was an *assemblage* of antique cars.
al	related to; process of	His *approval* rating was the lowest ever obtained.
ance	condition of	The building was not in *compliance* with city codes.
ate	having	Church members would *alienate* divorced couples.
ation	process of; action	The *publication* date was set for the end of the month.

Table 3.2
Common Suffixes

Suffix	Meaning	Example
cy	condition of; state of	*Vagrancy* was a problem for the city.
ed	past tense of a verb	The child *walked* five miles to go fishing.
en	to cause to be	The father carved a *wooden* horse for his daughter's birthday present.
ence	state of; condition of	People should value their *independence*.
er	one who performs	Everyone said she should be a *teacher*.
ery	state of; place	The nurse worked in *surgery*.
ese	quality of	The restaurant served *Chinese* food.
ia, ial	pertaining to	The student read the *tutorial* for the program.
ian	related to; belonging to	Her secretary was the *historian* for the city.
ing	action	*Running* the mile in less than six minutes was her goal.
ist	one who performs an action	The orchestra had a violin *soloist*.
ious	full of; having	The deacon was a *religious* man.
ish	characteristic of	Children often act *foolish*.
ism	action; quality of	*Alcoholism* is a serious problem in some segments of society.
ity	action; process of	There was one *abnormality* in the test results.
ive	performing an action	The couple had an *abusive* relationship.
ize	to cause to be	Instructions said to *sterilize* the instruments.
less	without	The procedure was advertised as a *bloodless* surgery.
logy	study of	*Biology* is required for a high school diploma.
ment	action; process of	The coat was a *replacement* for the one he lost.
meter	measurement of	The *thermometer* indicated the patient's temperature was above normal.
ness	quality; condition	Male pattern *baldness* is a problem for some men.
oid	resembling	The being had *humanoid* qualities.
or	state of	Her child's *behavior* was offensive.

Table 3.2
Common Suffixes

Suffix	Meaning	Example
ory	characterized by	The church's *advisory* committee voted against a raise in pay for the minister.
ose	full of; possessing	After being hit on the head, the man was *comatose*.
osis	condition	*Osmosis* is the dispersion of fluid through a semipermeable membrane.
s, es	plural of a noun; more than one	Ten *drivers* registered for the race.
ship	state of; quality of	Their *friendship* had lasted for years.
some	full of	The police made a *gruesome* discovery.
tion	action; condition of	The minister gave the *benediction*.
ty	quality; condition of	Singing is an *activity* enjoyed by children.

Root Words

Root words are words that communicate the fundamental meaning of a particular word. Root words form the nucleus of a word and are the basis for words in a language. Prefixes and suffixes are combined with or attached to these words to create other words or to change the meaning of the root words. Some words are combinations of more than one root word and are used to create another word that may have a similar or completely opposite meaning.

A partial list of root words follows in Table 3.3. Consult a dictionary for more root words.

Table 3.3
Common Root Words

Root	Meaning	Example
ac	to do	No *action* was taken against the trespassers.
ag	to do	The secretary read the *agenda* to the committee members.
agri	farm	Her college major was *agribusiness*.
anthropo	man	*Anthropology* is the study of man.
aqua	water	The new swimming pool was called the *aquatic* center.
aud	hearing	*Audiovisuals* enhanced the student's difficult presentation.
auto	self	The car had an *automatic* transmission.

Table 3.3
Common Root Words

Root	Meaning	Example
biblio	book	A *bibliography* or reference section is at the end of the paper.
bio	life	The actor completed his *autobiography* two weeks ago.
cad	fall	The drum *cadence* could be heard for blocks.
capit	head	Austin is the *capital* of Texas.
cede	go	The parents needed to *intercede* with their children.
celer	speed	He pushed the car's *accelerator* to the floor.
chron	time	A *chronograph* recorded the duration of the event.
cide	kill; cut	The gardener sprayed an *insecticide* on the trees.
clude	close	Adults did not want to *include* the children.
cog	know; knowledge	Our psychologist tested the child's *cognitive* abilities.
ded	give	The *dedication* for the monument was scheduled for next week.
dent	tooth	The child needed a *dental* appointment.
duc	lead	The adult could not *induce* the child to take the money.
fac	make; do	Our company *manufactured* leather shoes.
fer	carry	The nurse *transferred* to another floor.
fract	break	The child *fractured* his arm when he fell.
frater	brother	He wanted to join a *fraternity*.
gen	produce	The job would *generate* money for the family.
geo	earth	Children learn about different countries in *geography* class.
graph	picture; writing	The couple bought software containing computer *graphics*.
hemo	blood	The woman's *hemoglobin* was lower than normal.
homo	man	The police investigated the *homicide*.
hydr	water	The dam produced *hydroelectricity*.
ject	throw	A child was *rejected* by his friends.
jud	right	The *judge* suspended the sentence and freed the man.
junct	join	A *conjunction* is a part of speech.
juris	justice; law	This crime occurred outside of the police department's *jurisdiction*.

Table 3.3
Common Root Words

Root	Meaning	Example
lect	read	The *lecture* lasted for an hour.
logue	speech	Her *dialogue* confused the students who had not read the material.
loq	speak	The author was an *eloquent* speaker.
lude	play	The *interlude* lasted for fifteen minutes.
manu	hand	The old *manuscript* was written by Aristotle.
mand	order	The major was the *commander* of the unit.
mater	mother	The woman was his *maternal* grandmother.
mort	death	A *mortician* prepared the body for the funeral.
mute	change	A judge *commuted* the sentence.
naut	sailor; ship	The islands were ten *nautical* miles apart.
nounce	declare	The judge *announced* the winners of the games.
ped	foot	The teenager thought her feet would look better after a *pedicure*.
philo	love	A young student studied *philosophy* as an undergraduate.
port	carry	The woman took her *portable* radio to the park.
psych	mind	He studied to be a clinical *psychologist*.
reg	rule	The company had many *regulations*.
rupt	break	Children *disrupted* the game.
sect	cut	Students taking gross anatomy *dissect* cadavers.
sert	bind	The missing pages were *inserted* into the manuscript.
scend	climb	The man fell while *descending* the ladder.
scribe	write	The jeweler *inscribed*, "To my husband of fifty wonderful years," on the plaque.
spect	look at	The man was a *spectator* at all of his son's football games.
spir	breath	The *respiratory* rate of an infant is faster than that of an adult.
strict	tighten	There were no *restrictions* on travel.
tain	hold	The woman asked for a one-quart *container*.
term	end	His business *terminated* the contract.
tract	draw	The car's wheels had little *traction* on the ice.
typ	print	Most students would rather use a word processor than a *typewriter*.

Table 3.3
Common Root Words

Root	Meaning	Example
ven	come	The meeting *convened* at dusk.
vict	conquer	The football team had a *victorious* season.
vis	see	The child needed a *visual* exam because he was seeing double.
volt	turn	Soldiers *revolted* against the king.

Antonyms and Synonyms

Words are more than their parts—prefixes, roots, and suffixes. They have meanings. Numerous words have almost the same or identical meanings, and many other words are opposite in meaning. These are the synonyms and antonyms.

Using antonyms and synonyms can enhance your written and verbal communication with others. Listening to or writing the same word or words again and again is repetitive, and suggests that your vocabulary may be limited. Your reader or listener may lose interest when you use the same word or words repeatedly.

Antonyms are words that are opposite in meaning. Words such as hot and cold, happy and sad, young and old, good and bad, and inside and outside are antonyms. Antonyms do not reveal the degree or condition of the word. Take hot and cold water for example; the words *hot* and *cold* do not tell us how hot or how cold the water actually is. They only tell us the relative temperature of the water.

Synonyms are often thought of as being the opposite of antonyms; they are words that are identical or almost the same in meaning. Words such as audacity and boldness, bondage and slavery, nomad and wanderer, hazard and danger, and ingenious and clever are synonyms. Like antonyms, synonyms do not indicate the degree or amount. The words hazard and danger suggest a potential for injury in a given situation, but how hazardous or how dangerous a situation is cannot be determined from the words alone.

Antonym and synonym sample tests with answer sheets and answer keys follow. You will learn more if you take the test before looking at the answer key. When selecting answers using a multiple-choice format, make sure that you determine why each response is right or wrong. Good test takers know why a response is right as well as why the remaining responses are wrong.

Answer Sheet
SAMPLE TEST ONE

Antonym

1 Ⓐ Ⓑ Ⓒ Ⓓ
2 Ⓐ Ⓑ Ⓒ Ⓓ
3 Ⓐ Ⓑ Ⓒ Ⓓ
4 Ⓐ Ⓑ Ⓒ Ⓓ
5 Ⓐ Ⓑ Ⓒ Ⓓ
6 Ⓐ Ⓑ Ⓒ Ⓓ
7 Ⓐ Ⓑ Ⓒ Ⓓ
8 Ⓐ Ⓑ Ⓒ Ⓓ
9 Ⓐ Ⓑ Ⓒ Ⓓ

10 Ⓐ Ⓑ Ⓒ Ⓓ
11 Ⓐ Ⓑ Ⓒ Ⓓ
12 Ⓐ Ⓑ Ⓒ Ⓓ
13 Ⓐ Ⓑ Ⓒ Ⓓ
14 Ⓐ Ⓑ Ⓒ Ⓓ
15 Ⓐ Ⓑ Ⓒ Ⓓ
16 Ⓐ Ⓑ Ⓒ Ⓓ
17 Ⓐ Ⓑ Ⓒ Ⓓ
18 Ⓐ Ⓑ Ⓒ Ⓓ

19 Ⓐ Ⓑ Ⓒ Ⓓ
20 Ⓐ Ⓑ Ⓒ Ⓓ
21 Ⓐ Ⓑ Ⓒ Ⓓ
22 Ⓐ Ⓑ Ⓒ Ⓓ
23 Ⓐ Ⓑ Ⓒ Ⓓ
24 Ⓐ Ⓑ Ⓒ Ⓓ
25 Ⓐ Ⓑ Ⓒ Ⓓ

Antonym Sample Test One

Directions: For each of the numbered pairs of words, select the letter (A, B, C, or D) in which the paired words are *opposite* in meaning. Record your answers on the answer sheet on page 43.

1. (A) Teach - Learn
   (B) Counter - Workbench
   (C) Conceal - Camouflage
   (D) Offensive - Distasteful

2. (A) Obesity - Adiposity
   (B) Nag - Nuisance
   (C) Specific - Indefinite
   (D) Adherence - Association

3. (A) Deceptive - Misleading
   (B) Vulnerable - Susceptible
   (C) Durable - Impermanent
   (D) Solitude - Seclusion

4. (A) Frugal - Spartan   **CHALLENGE**
   (B) Recant - Take back
   (C) Turgid - Swollen
   (D) Wicked - Innocent

5. (A) Secret - Open
   (B) Indictment - Charge
   (C) Hollow - Vacuous
   (D) Hectic - Chaotic

6. (A) Laudable - Praiseworthy
   (B) Deplete - Hoard
   (C) Prior - Former
   (D) Ability - Aptitude

7. (A) Include - Exclude
   (B) Later - Subsequent
   (C) Eager - Ardent
   (D) Discipline - Correction

8. (A) Private - Known
   (B) Diligent - Industrious
   (C) Prolific - Fruitful
   (D) Replete - Full

9. (A) Absolve - Pardon
   (B) Inept - Adroit
   (C) Compliant - Submissive
   (D) Affinity - Rapport

10. (A) Nullify - Abolish   **CHALLENGE**
    (B) Acrimony - Irascibility
    (C) Concur - Agree
    (D) Abstinent - Insatiable

11. (A) Ardor - Fervor
    (B) Blunt - Sharp
    (C) Cauterize - Burn
    (D) Bovine - Cowlike

12. (A) Sloth - Laziness
    (B) Avarice - Greed
    (C) Amenable - Opposing
    (D) Commodious - Roomy

13. (A) Retard - Hasten
    (B) Germane - Relevant
    (C) Solemn - Grave
    (D) Appraise - Estimate

14. (A) Scorn - Mock
    (B) Fauna - Flora
    (C) Pretend - Concoct
    (D) Fetish - Amulet

15. (A) Candid - Frank
    (B) Happy - Merry
    (C) Avoid - Shun
    (D) Impudent - Courteous

16. (A) Flagon - Flask
    (B) Precipitous - Steep
    (C) Humble - Pompous
    (D) Peruse - Study

17. (A) Sequester - Set apart   CHALLENGE
    (B) Tepid - Lukewarm
    (C) Stringent - Lax
    (D) Wan - Sickly

18. (A) Homogeneous - Uniform
    (B) Proscribe - Outlaw
    (C) Venial - Forgivable
    (D) Morbid - Wholesome

19. (A) False - Forged
    (B) Boorish - Urbane
    (C) Surmise - Imagine
    (D) Temerity - Audacity

20. (A) Flux - Change
    (B) Perfidy - Fidelity
    (C) Stealthy - Shifty
    (D) Gregarious - Sociable

21. (A) Alms - Charity
    (B) Dauntless - Fearless
    (C) Hood - Cowl
    (D) Impromptu - Planned

22. (A) Judicious - Imprudent
    (B) Flaccid - Limp
    (C) Hirsute - Hairy
    (D) Gulch - Ravine

23. (A) Pariah - Outcast
    (B) Tawdry - Cheap
    (C) Inept - Dexterous
    (D) Terse - Concise

24. (A) Tacit - Explicit
    (B) Flaunt - Exhibit
    (C) Illicit - Unlawful
    (D) Flammable - Combustible

25. (A) Windward - Leeward
    (B) Harsh - Grating
    (C) Revile - Scold
    (D) Quell - Suppress

Antonym Sample Test One Answer Key

1. **(A)**	6. **(B)**	11. **(B)**	16. **(C)**	21. **(D)**
2. **(C)**	7. **(A)**	12. **(C)**	17. **(C)**	22. **(A)**
3. **(C)**	8. **(A)**	13. **(A)**	18. **(D)**	23. **(C)**
4. **(D)**	9. **(B)**	14. **(B)**	19. **(B)**	24. **(A)**
5. **(A)**	10. **(D)**	15. **(D)**	20. **(B)**	25. **(A)**

Answer Sheet
SAMPLE TEST TWO

Antonym

1 Ⓐ Ⓑ Ⓒ Ⓓ	10 Ⓐ Ⓑ Ⓒ Ⓓ	19 Ⓐ Ⓑ Ⓒ Ⓓ
2 Ⓐ Ⓑ Ⓒ Ⓓ	11 Ⓐ Ⓑ Ⓒ Ⓓ	20 Ⓐ Ⓑ Ⓒ Ⓓ
3 Ⓐ Ⓑ Ⓒ Ⓓ	12 Ⓐ Ⓑ Ⓒ Ⓓ	21 Ⓐ Ⓑ Ⓒ Ⓓ
4 Ⓐ Ⓑ Ⓒ Ⓓ	13 Ⓐ Ⓑ Ⓒ Ⓓ	22 Ⓐ Ⓑ Ⓒ Ⓓ
5 Ⓐ Ⓑ Ⓒ Ⓓ	14 Ⓐ Ⓑ Ⓒ Ⓓ	23 Ⓐ Ⓑ Ⓒ Ⓓ
6 Ⓐ Ⓑ Ⓒ Ⓓ	15 Ⓐ Ⓑ Ⓒ Ⓓ	24 Ⓐ Ⓑ Ⓒ Ⓓ
7 Ⓐ Ⓑ Ⓒ Ⓓ	16 Ⓐ Ⓑ Ⓒ Ⓓ	25 Ⓐ Ⓑ Ⓒ Ⓓ
8 Ⓐ Ⓑ Ⓒ Ⓓ	17 Ⓐ Ⓑ Ⓒ Ⓓ	
9 Ⓐ Ⓑ Ⓒ Ⓓ	18 Ⓐ Ⓑ Ⓒ Ⓓ	

Antonyms Sample Test Two

Antonym Sample Test Two

Directions: For each of the numbered words, select the letter (A, B, C, or D) in which the paired words is *opposite* in meaning. Record your answers on the answer sheet on page 47.

1. Rigid

   (A) Format
   (B) Right
   (C) Yielding
   (D) Rickety

2. Modern

   (A) Avant-garde
   (B) Antiquated
   (C) Impact
   (D) Kind

3. Archaic

   (A) Arch
   (B) Medieval
   (C) Lightning
   (D) Young

4. Refuse

   (A) Accept
   (B) Spurn
   (C) Garbage
   (D) Regain

5. Announce

   (A) Forswear
   (B) Dovetail
   (C) Conceal
   (D) Drive

6. Cunning

   (A) Naive
   (B) Exact
   (C) Smart
   (D) Trustworthy

7. Unforeseen

   (A) Predictable
   (B) Umbrage
   (C) Undulate
   (D) Marginal

8. Shape

   (A) Round
   (B) Tighten
   (C) Destroy
   (D) Empower

9. Impair

   (A) Pair
   (B) Aid
   (C) Nullify
   (D) Compendious

10. Flex

    (A) Reflex
    (B) Tighten
    (C) Weight
    (D) Extend

11. Boil

    (A) Anger
    (B) Material
    (C) Enrapture
    (D) Assuage

12. Defective

    (A) Faultless
    (B) Police
    (C) Reject
    (D) Rejoin

13. Inhospitable

    (A) Corrupt
    (B) Askew
    (C) Genial
    (D) Independence

14. Sever

    (A) Cut
    (B) Associate
    (C) Hard
    (D) Nourish

15. Charge

    (A) Rent
    (B) Rotate
    (C) Chemical
    (D) Absolve

16. Rehabilitate

    (A) Walk
    (B) Investigate
    (C) Destroy
    (D) Comprehensive

17. Manifest `CHALLENGE`

    (A) Invaluable
    (B) Unclear
    (C) Natural
    (D) Developing

18. Fertile

    (A) Crescent
    (B) Soil
    (C) Gestation
    (D) Unproductive

19. Felicitous

    (A) Improper
    (B) Catlike
    (C) Mourning
    (D) Defeat

20. Cordial

    (A) Party
    (B) Unsociable
    (C) Headstrong
    (D) Enjoyable

21. Rupture

    (A) Heaven
    (B) Torn
    (C) Mend
    (D) Elastic

22. Strong `CHALLENGE`

    (A) Chary
    (B) Irresolute
    (C) Overwrought
    (D) Incline

23. Impasse

    (A) Parch
    (B) Destroy
    (C) Flow
    (D) Agreement

24. Torpid `CHALLENGE`

    (A) Kidnap
    (B) Compliant
    (C) Essential
    (D) Energetic

25. Crude

    (A) Polished
    (B) Rough
    (C) Gasoline
    (D) Graded

Antonym Sample Test Two Answer Key

1. (C)	6. (A)	11. (D)	16. (C)	21. (C)
2. (B)	7. (A)	12. (A)	17. (B)	22. (B)
3. (D)	8. (C)	13. (C)	18. (D)	23. (D)
4. (A)	9. (B)	14. (B)	19. (A)	24. (D)
5. (C)	10. (D)	15. (D)	20. (B)	25. (A)

Antonyms Sample Test Two

Answer Sheet
SAMPLE TEST ONE

Synonym

1 Ⓐ Ⓑ Ⓒ Ⓓ   10 Ⓐ Ⓑ Ⓒ Ⓓ   19 Ⓐ Ⓑ Ⓒ Ⓓ
2 Ⓐ Ⓑ Ⓒ Ⓓ   11 Ⓐ Ⓑ Ⓒ Ⓓ   20 Ⓐ Ⓑ Ⓒ Ⓓ
3 Ⓐ Ⓑ Ⓒ Ⓓ   12 Ⓐ Ⓑ Ⓒ Ⓓ   21 Ⓐ Ⓑ Ⓒ Ⓓ
4 Ⓐ Ⓑ Ⓒ Ⓓ   13 Ⓐ Ⓑ Ⓒ Ⓓ   22 Ⓐ Ⓑ Ⓒ Ⓓ
5 Ⓐ Ⓑ Ⓒ Ⓓ   14 Ⓐ Ⓑ Ⓒ Ⓓ   23 Ⓐ Ⓑ Ⓒ Ⓓ
6 Ⓐ Ⓑ Ⓒ Ⓓ   15 Ⓐ Ⓑ Ⓒ Ⓓ   24 Ⓐ Ⓑ Ⓒ Ⓓ
7 Ⓐ Ⓑ Ⓒ Ⓓ   16 Ⓐ Ⓑ Ⓒ Ⓓ   25 Ⓐ Ⓑ Ⓒ Ⓓ
8 Ⓐ Ⓑ Ⓒ Ⓓ   17 Ⓐ Ⓑ Ⓒ Ⓓ
9 Ⓐ Ⓑ Ⓒ Ⓓ   18 Ⓐ Ⓑ Ⓒ Ⓓ

Synonym Sample Test One

Directions: For each of the numbered words, select the letter (A, B, C, or D) in which the word is the *same* or *almost the same* in meaning. Record your answers on the answer sheet on page 51.

1. (A) Defend - Abandon
   (B) Portent - Marvel
   (C) Applaud - Decry
   (D) Reflect - Dismiss

2. (A) Ubiquitous - Everywhere   CHALLENGE
   (B) Curl - Straighten
   (C) Odious - Kind
   (D) Bizarre - Conventional

3. (A) Incomplete - Fully
   (B) Umbrage - Anger
   (C) Estranged - Friendly
   (D) Following - Ahead

4. (A) Blighted - Blessed
   (B) Attach - Unconfined
   (C) Sweet - Biting
   (D) Posterity - Children

5. (A) Barbarous - Civilized
   (B) Whimper - Howl
   (C) Impeach - Accuse
   (D) Whet - Dull

6. (A) Twilight - Daybreak
   (B) Vacant - Overflowing
   (C) Forswear - Abandon
   (D) Valiant - Timid

7. (A) Yearn - Ache
   (B) Blur - Clear
   (C) Bloom - Shrink
   (D) Harebrained - Wise

8. (A) Dour - Bright
   (B) Attest - Deny
   (C) Tenacious - Sticky
   (D) Intuitive - Calculate

9. (A) Corrode - Build
   (B) Whitewash - Camouflage
   (C) Copious - Lacking
   (D) Board - Evict

10. (A) Pout - Grin
    (B) Mar - Heal
    (C) Sweet - Rancid
    (D) Allege - Adduce

11. (A) Roll - Steady
    (B) Malign - Blacken
    (C) Like - Diverse
    (D) Dolt - Brain

12. (A) Paraphrase - Restate
    (B) Smooth - Wrinkle
    (C) Enormous - Minute
    (D) Complicated - Easy

13. (A) Think - Disbelieve
    (B) Maritime - Aquatic
    (C) Struggle - Idle
    (D) Stint - Spend

14. (A) Sore - Happy
    (B) Spare - Condemn
    (C) Douse - Deluge
    (D) Abscond - Offer

15. (A) Robust - Flabby
    (B) Calm - Rouse
    (C) Quack - Genuine
    (D) Cooperative - Obliging

16. (A) Puzzle - Clarify   CHALLENGE
    (B) Cosmetic - Corrective
    (C) Promiscuous - Temperate
    (D) Downsize - Augment

17. (A) Verdant - Flourishing
    (B) Flaccid - Firm
    (C) Lavish - Economize
    (D) Admonish - Laud

18. (A) Abide - Vacate
    (B) Theological - Secular
    (C) Vibration - Beating
    (D) Dramatic - Straight

19. (A) Oaf - Sage
    (B) August - Common
    (C) Spawn - Create
    (D) Executive - Underling

20. (A) Ghastly - Pleasing
    (B) Reflect - Absorb
    (C) Rough - Nice
    (D) Boisterous - Clamorous

21. (A) Consummate - Begin
    (B) Burrow - Cover
    (C) Flighty - Steady
    (D) Catholic - Broad

22. (A) Censure - Berate
    (B) Ace - Inept
    (C) Flux - Stability
    (D) Impertinent - Civil

23. (A) Covet - Abjure
    (B) Deep - Abysmal
    (C) Defeat - Give up
    (D) Fine - Award

24. (A) Curtail - Extend
    (B) Limber - Tense
    (C) Drudge - Dig
    (D) Desecrate - Honor

25. (A) Immune - Subject
    (B) Mollify - Abate
    (C) Ludicrous - Logical
    (D) Rank - Scatter

Synonym Sample Test One Answer Key

1. **(B)**	6. **(C)**	11. **(B)**	16. **(B)**	21. **(D)**
2. **(A)**	7. **(A)**	12. **(A)**	17. **(A)**	22. **(A)**
3. **(B)**	8. **(C)**	13. **(B)**	18. **(C)**	23. **(B)**
4. **(D)**	9. **(B)**	14. **(C)**	19. **(C)**	24. **(C)**
5. **(C)**	10. **(D)**	15. **(D)**	20. **(D)**	25. **(B)**

Answer Sheet
SAMPLE TEST TWO

Synonym

1 Ⓐ Ⓑ Ⓒ Ⓓ	10 Ⓐ Ⓑ Ⓒ Ⓓ	19 Ⓐ Ⓑ Ⓒ Ⓓ
2 Ⓐ Ⓑ Ⓒ Ⓓ	11 Ⓐ Ⓑ Ⓒ Ⓓ	20 Ⓐ Ⓑ Ⓒ Ⓓ
3 Ⓐ Ⓑ Ⓒ Ⓓ	12 Ⓐ Ⓑ Ⓒ Ⓓ	21 Ⓐ Ⓑ Ⓒ Ⓓ
4 Ⓐ Ⓑ Ⓒ Ⓓ	13 Ⓐ Ⓑ Ⓒ Ⓓ	22 Ⓐ Ⓑ Ⓒ Ⓓ
5 Ⓐ Ⓑ Ⓒ Ⓓ	14 Ⓐ Ⓑ Ⓒ Ⓓ	23 Ⓐ Ⓑ Ⓒ Ⓓ
6 Ⓐ Ⓑ Ⓒ Ⓓ	15 Ⓐ Ⓑ Ⓒ Ⓓ	24 Ⓐ Ⓑ Ⓒ Ⓓ
7 Ⓐ Ⓑ Ⓒ Ⓓ	16 Ⓐ Ⓑ Ⓒ Ⓓ	25 Ⓐ Ⓑ Ⓒ Ⓓ
8 Ⓐ Ⓑ Ⓒ Ⓓ	17 Ⓐ Ⓑ Ⓒ Ⓓ	
9 Ⓐ Ⓑ Ⓒ Ⓓ	18 Ⓐ Ⓑ Ⓒ Ⓓ	

Answer Sheet

SAMPLE TEST TWO

Synonyms

Synonym Sample Test Two

Directions: For each of the numbered words, select the letter (A, B, C, or D) in which the word is the *same* or *almost the same* in meaning. Record your answers on the answer sheet on page 55.

1. Abstruse   CHALLENGE

   (A) Instruct
   (B) Obscure
   (C) Obtuse
   (D) Rigging

2. Nimble

   (A) Skillful
   (B) Simple
   (C) Personal
   (D) Historical

3. Adversary

   (A) Averse
   (B) Caution
   (C) Opponent
   (D) Zeal

4. Oblivion

   (A) Forgetfulness
   (B) Avarice
   (C) Profess
   (D) Fatal

5. Opulence

   (A) Inane
   (B) Chandelier
   (C) Sagacious
   (D) Luxuriousness

6. Muted

   (A) Initiate
   (B) Silent
   (C) Oversight
   (D) Enrage

7. Plight

   (A) Condition
   (B) Hinder
   (C) Imprison
   (D) Minor

8. Disputatious   CHALLENGE

   (A) Polemical
   (B) Immutable
   (C) Iconoclast
   (D) Motive

9. Combativeness

   (A) Malign
   (B) Bungling
   (C) Pugnacity
   (D) Obedient

10. Reticent

    (A) Disfigured
    (B) Reserved
    (C) Lucid
    (D) Graphic

11. Rudimentary

    (A) Offensive
    (B) Peripheral
    (C) Tedium
    (D) Elementary

12. Tyranny

    (A) Suspend
    (B) Dinosaur
    (C) Turbulence
    (D) Oppression

13. Virulent

(A) Defective
(B) Violent
(C) Hostile
(D) Fallacious

14. Magnanimous

(A) Exuberance
(B) Generous
(C) Comprehensive
(D) Vanishing

15. Wind

(A) Extol
(B) Disentangle
(C) Meander
(D) Extreme

16. Lassitude

(A) Embitter
(B) Adopt
(C) Robust
(D) Languor

17. Indubitable **CHALLENGE**

(A) Unquestionable
(B) Irreverence
(C) Threatening
(D) Stupid

18. Hone

(A) Dark
(B) Sharpen
(C) Dwelling
(D) Nebulous

19. Blessed

(A) Naiveté
(B) Wicked
(C) Worldly
(D) Hallowed

20. Germane

(A) Pertinent
(B) Foreign
(C) Stubborn
(D) Trite

21. Founder

(A) Vertebrate
(B) Condition
(C) Sink
(D) Insightful

22. Garbled

(A) Biased
(B) Marginal
(C) Jumbled
(D) Pliant

23. Innocuous

(A) Commonplace
(B) Harmless
(C) Hedonist
(D) Sneaky

24. Dull

(A) Obstruct
(B) Disoriented
(C) Duplicity
(D) Insipid

25. Ephemeral **CHALLENGE**

(A) Arrogance
(B) Fruitless
(C) Encourage
(D) Fleeting

Synonym Sample Test Two Answer Key

1. **(B)**	6. **(B)**	11. **(D)**	16. **(D)**	21. **(C)**
2. **(A)**	7. **(A)**	12. **(D)**	17. **(A)**	22. **(C)**
3. **(C)**	8. **(A)**	13. **(C)**	18. **(B)**	23. **(B)**
4. **(A)**	9. **(C)**	14. **(B)**	19. **(D)**	24. **(D)**
5. **(D)**	10. **(B)**	15. **(C)**	20. **(A)**	25. **(D)**

Analogies

Verbal analogies are word problems based on logical assumptions and are an indicator of an individual's ability to analyze, think, and reason critically. The capacity to perform these higher-level tasks is related to intelligence.

Verbal Analogy Format

Verbal analogies are presented like proportion problems commonly found in math or algebra. Analogies may be presented in one of five different formats. In each format, a missing term or terms must be furnished.

EXAMPLE OF FORMAT ONE

BIG : LITTLE :: _____
(A) GREEN : APPLE
(B) ROAD : CAR
(C) FISH : FISHERMAN
(D) FAT : SKINNY

The correct answer is FAT : SKINNY, choice D. The problem can be solved utilizing two different approaches. By looking at the relationships between the words, you can see that BIG and LITTLE are antonyms as are FAT and SKINNY. You can also see that BIG and FAT are synonyms as are LITTLE and SKINNY.

EXAMPLE OF FORMAT TWO

_____ : LITTLE :: FAT : SKINNY
(A) ROMANCE
(B) LARGE
(C) BIG
(D) PILLOW

The correct answer is BIG, choice C. The same reasoning used to solve Format One is used to solve Format Two.

EXAMPLE OF FORMAT THREE

BIG : _____ :: FAT : SKINNY
(A) MOUNTAIN
(B) BIGGER
(C) PAPER
(D) LITTLE

The correct answer is LITTLE, choice D.

EXAMPLE OF FORMAT FOUR

BIG : LITTLE :: _____ : SKINNY
(A) FAT
(B) THIN
(C) MONDO
(D) FISH

The correct answer is FAT, choice A.

EXAMPLE OF FORMAT FIVE

BIG : LITTLE :: FAT : _____
(A) OBESE
(B) OBSESSIVE
(C) IMPORTANT
(D) SKINNY

The correct answer is SKINNY, choice D.

Verbal Analogy Content

Verbal analogies are grouped according to subject matter or content. Content areas include the social and natural sciences, mathematics, humanities, commonplace information, and English grammar, usage, and vocabulary. Here is an example of each.

SOCIAL SCIENCE EXAMPLE

DEMOCRACY : BY THE PEOPLE :: _____ : STATE RULE
(A) FRANCHISE
(B) JUNTA
(C) CHECKS AND BALANCES
(D) DICTATORSHIP

The correct answer is DICTATORSHIP, choice D. Both democracy and dictatorship are forms of government. In a democracy, the government is by the people. In a dictatorship, the government is state ruled by an individual with strict power and authority.

NATURAL SCIENCES EXAMPLE

DARWIN : EVOLUTION :: _____ : RELATIVITY
(A) GALILEO
(B) MENDEL
(C) EINSTEIN
(D) SALK

The correct answer is EINSTEIN, choice C. Darwin developed the theory of evolution; Einstein developed the theory of relativity.

MATHEMATICS EXAMPLE

_____ : 10, 14, 18 :: 2, 14, 26 : 6, 12, 18
(A) 11, 13, 15
(B) −2, 2, 6
(C) 7, 15, 23
(D) 3, 13, 23

The correct answer is 7, 15, 23, choice C, where 7 + 8 = 15 + 8 = 23. Each number is larger by 8. In the second set of numbers (10, 14, 18), 10 + 4 = 14 + 4 = 18. Each number is larger by four. In the third series of numbers (2, 14, 26), 2 + 12 = 14 + 12 = 26. Each number is larger by 12. In the final series of numbers (6, 12, 18), 6 + 6 = 12 + 6 = 18. Each number is larger by 6 or half the amount in the previous series where each number is larger by 12. In looking at the possible answers, only option C is reasonable. The increase in the first series of numbers (7, 15, 23) is double the increase of the second series of numbers (10, 14, 18).

HUMANITIES EXAMPLE

PARABLE : MORAL TRUTH :: PARODY : _____
(A) RIDICULE
(B) ROMANTICIZE
(C) TRILOGY
(D) POLITICAL INSIGHT

The correct answer is RIDICULE, choice A. A parable is a story that portrays a moral truth or teaching. A parody is an amusing literary composition that makes fun of a serious literary work.

COMMONPLACE INFORMATION EXAMPLE

SHEEP : _____ :: SWAN : CYGNET
(A) VIXEN
(B) COB
(C) LAMB
(D) CALF

The correct answer is LAMB, choice C. The offspring of a ewe, a female sheep, is a lamb. The offspring of a swan is a cygnet.

ENGLISH GRAMMAR AND USAGE EXAMPLE

CONCRETE NOUN : CINNAMON :: _____ : FREEDOM
(A) COLLECTIVE NOUN
(B) COMMON NOUN
(C) PROPER NOUN
(D) ABSTRACT NOUN

The correct answer is ABSTRACT NOUN, chioce D. A concrete noun is one that can be perceived by the senses. Cinnamon has a distinctive aroma. An abstract noun is one that cannot be pictured or reasoned by the senses. Freedom is an abstract concept.

Verbal Analogy Relationship Patterns

Verbal analogies fall into a number of basic relationship patterns that require the test taker to recognize relationships between pairs of abstractions or ideas. Recognizing these relationships requires higher levels of reasoning and thinking. Here are some examples of the various types of relationship patterns.

PART TO WHOLE EXAMPLE

LEAD : PENCIL :: _____ : EYE
(A) SKULL
(B) REACTION
(C) IRIS
(D) SKIN

The correct answer is IRIS, choice C. Lead is a part of a pencil. The iris is a part of the eye.

WHOLE TO PART EXAMPLE

ENGINE : _____ :: FOOT : TOE
(A) CAR
(B) GASOLINE
(C) SPARK PLUG
(D) TIRE

The correct answer is SPARK PLUG, choice C. One of the parts of an engine is a spark plug. One of the parts of the foot is the toe.

SYNONYM EXAMPLE

PROCLIVITY : INCLINATION :: BARBAROUS : _____
(A) UNCOUTH
(B) REFINED
(C) TYPICAL
(D) VOLATILE

The correct answer is UNCOUTH, choice A. Barbarous and uncouth are synonyms, as are proclivity and inclination.

ANTONYM EXAMPLE

ATTENUATE : INTENSIFY :: _____ : _____
(A) EFFETE : EXHAUSTED
(B) POLTROON : COWARD
(C) RUMINATE : PONDER
(D) VERBOSE : LACONIC

The correct answer is VERBOSE : LACONIC, choice D. Verbose also means wordy or long-winded; laconic means brief or to the point. The words are antonyms.

CAUSE AND EFFECT EXAMPLE

RAIN : FLOOD :: _____ : DEATH
(A) TRUMP
(B) HEMORRHAGE
(C) NIGHT
(D) WINTER

The correct answer is HEMORRHAGE, choice B. Too much rain can cause a flood. Too much hemorrhage, or uncontrolled bleeding, can cause death.

DEGREE EXAMPLE

DECIBEL : SOUND :: _____ : EARTHQUAKE
(A) RIPPLES
(B) METRONOME
(C) MAGNITUDE
(D) QUIVER

The correct answer is MAGNITUDE, choice C. Decibels are units used to express differences in loudness or softness of sound. Earthquakes are measured in terms of their magnitude.

DEFINING CHARACTERISTIC EXAMPLE

CLAWS : CAT :: _____ : HORSE
(A) FOOT
(B) HOOVES
(C) STAG
(D) SPINE

The correct answer is HOOVES, choice B. A cat by definition has claws; horses have hooves.

SEQUENCE EXAMPLE

_____ : BIRTH :: BUD : FLOWER
(A) DEATH
(B) ABSTINENCE
(C) CONCEPTION
(D) LEAF

The correct answer is CONCEPTION, choice C. Conception takes place before birth can occur, and a bud develops before a flower blooms.

GENDER EXAMPLES

BULL : _____ :: ROOSTER : CAPON
(A) GELDING
(B) BUCK
(C) STEER
(D) COW

The correct answer is STEER, choice C. A castrated bull is referred to as a steer. A castrated rooster is referred to as a capon.

Analogy sample tests with answer sheets and answer keys follow. As with previous tests you will learn more if you answer the questions before looking at the answer key. Make sure that you determine why each response is right or wrong. Remember that good test takers know why a response is right as well as why the remaining responses are wrong.

Answer Sheet
SAMPLE TEST ONE

Analogy

1 (A) (B) (C) (D)
2 (A) (B) (C) (D)
3 (A) (B) (C) (D)
4 (A) (B) (C) (D)
5 (A) (B) (C) (D)
6 (A) (B) (C) (D)
7 (A) (B) (C) (D)
8 (A) (B) (C) (D)
9 (A) (B) (C) (D)

10 (A) (B) (C) (D)
11 (A) (B) (C) (D)
12 (A) (B) (C) (D)
13 (A) (B) (C) (D)
14 (A) (B) (C) (D)
15 (A) (B) (C) (D)
16 (A) (B) (C) (D)
17 (A) (B) (C) (D)
18 (A) (B) (C) (D)

19 (A) (B) (C) (D)
20 (A) (B) (C) (D)
21 (A) (B) (C) (D)
22 (A) (B) (C) (D)
23 (A) (B) (C) (D)
24 (A) (B) (C) (D)
25 (A) (B) (C) (D)

Analogy Sample Test One

Directions: For each of the questions, select the letter (A, B, C, or D) that makes the best match with the remaining analogous terms. Record your answers on the answer sheet on page 67.

1. RADISH : GARDEN :: _____ : ORCHARD

   (A) TULIP
   (B) GREEN BEAN
   (C) ROSE
   (D) APPLE

2. WE : PERSONAL PRONOUN :: MYSELF : _____

   (A) RELATIVE PRONOUN
   (B) INTERROGATIVE PRONOUN
   (C) INDEFINITE PRONOUN
   (D) REFLEXIVE PRONOUN

3. _____ : _____ :: 4, 6, 8, 10 : COMPOSITE NUMBERS

   (A) 2, 3, 5, 7 : PRIME NUMBERS   CHALLENGE
   (B) 1, 4, 6, 7 : RATIONAL NUMBERS
   (C) –3, –2, –1, 0 : NEGATIVE NUMBERS
   (D) 2, 2, 2, 2 : SQUARE NUMBERS

4. SHAKESPEARE : _____ :: HOMER : *THE ODYSSEY*

   (A) *STOPPING BY WOODS ON A SNOWY EVENING*
   (B) *GREAT EXPECTATIONS*
   (C) *HAMLET*
   (D) *THE RANSOM OF RED CHIEF*

5. PORTION : COLLECTION :: _____ : POWDERY

   (A) SANDY
   (B) SOLID
   (C) GRITTY
   (D) HOLD

6. FAMILY : _____ :: GENUS : HOMO

   (A) SAPIENS
   (B) CHORDATA
   (C) ANIMALIA
   (D) HOMINIDAE

7. ANTIETAM : SHILOH :: BUNKER HILL : _____

   (A) VALLEY FORGE
   (B) GETTYSBURG
   (C) VERDUN
   (D) DUNKIRK

8. GAGGLE : _____ :: SWARM : BEES

   (A) SWANS
   (B) PUPPIES
   (C) SNAILS
   (D) GEESE

9. SURNAME : FAMILY NAME :: _____ : PEN NAME

   (A) ANCESTOR
   (B) PSEUDONYM
   (C) PHILISTINE
   (D) BANAL

10. FLOUR : BREAD :: _____ : _____

   (A) IRIS : FRUIT
   (B) RUBBER : STRETCH
   (C) EGG : OMELET
   (D) THEATER : ARTS

11. ABIDE : _____ :: SLINK : SLUNK

   (A) ABODE
   (B) ABIDES
   (C) ABODEN
   (D) ABUDEN

12. ELECTRICAL SYSTEM : WIRES ::
    FLOWER : _____

    (A) SOIL
    (B) PETAL
    (C) ROSE
    (D) WATER

13. RUNNING : EXHAUSTION ::
    INFECTION : _____

    (A) WELLNESS
    (B) WOUND
    (C) VIRUS
    (D) FEVER

14. _____ : SLOW :: ALLEGRO : LIVELY

    (A) FUGUE
    (B) CODA
    (C) ADAGIO
    (D) FORTISSIMO

15. SUN : HEAT :: SKUNK : _____

    (A) NOCTURNAL
    (B) ODOR
    (C) ANIMAL
    (D) INVERTEBRATE

16. ENGAGED : MARRIAGE : _____ :
    DIVORCE

    (A) SEPARATION
    (B) ANNULMENT
    (C) AVAILABLE
    (D) REPULSIVE

17. DONNE : "DEATH BE NOT PROUD" ::
    _____ : "BECAUSE I COULD NOT
    STOP FOR DEATH"

    (A) DICKINSON
    (B) EMERSON
    (C) FROST
    (D) CLEMENS

18. PALEOZOIC ERA : _____ ::
    MESOZOIC ERA : MAMMALS

    (A) HUMANKIND   CHALLENGE
    (B) DINOSAURS
    (C) SPORES
    (D) FISHES

19. _____ : JUPITER :: HADES : PLUTO

    (A) VENUS
    (B) HERMES
    (C) ZEUS
    (D) APOLLO

20. ABSTRUSE : RUDIMENTARY ::
    ESOTERIC : _____

    (A) VORACIOUS   CHALLENGE
    (B) ELEMENTARY
    (C) RECONDITE
    (D) DEVOTION

21. AURORA BOREALIS : NORTHERN
    LIGHTS :: _____ : SOUTHERN
    LIGHTS

    (A) AURORA AUSTRALIS
    (B) AURORA ENNUE
    (C) AURORA GLISSANDO
    (D) AURORA GEOTROPISM

22. 100 METERS : HECTOMETER ::
    _____ : DECAMETER

    (A) 10,000 METERS   CHALLENGE
    (B) 1000 METERS
    (C) 10 METERS
    (D) 1 METER

23. HEART : CIRCULATION :: LUNGS :
    _____

    (A) GESTATION
    (B) DIGESTION
    (C) DECEREBRATION
    (D) OXYGENATION

24. PIAGET : INTELLECTUAL
    DEVELOPMENT :: _____ :
    MORAL DEVELOPMENT

    (A) JUNG
    (B) KOHLBERG
    (C) FREUD
    (D) PAVLOV

25. DECLARATION OF INDEPENDENCE :
    _____ :: THE U. S.
    CONSTITUTION : JAMES MADISON

    (A) ROGER WILLIAMS
    (B) THOMAS JEFFERSON
    (C) BRIGHAM YOUNG
    (D) ALEXANDER HAMILTON

Analogy Sample Test One Answer Key

1. **(D)** A radish is a vegetable, and vegetables are typically grown in a garden. An apple is a fruit, and fruits are typically grown in an orchard. Content area: Commonplace information.

2. **(D)** We is a personal pronoun; myself is a reflexive pronoun. Pronouns are words used in place of one or more nouns. *Content area:* English grammar, usage, and vocabulary.

3. **(A)** Prime numbers are numbers that can only be divided by themselves and 1. The numbers 2, 3, 5, and 7 are prime numbers. For example, 13 is a prime number that can evenly be divided by 13 and by 1 only. Composite numbers are divisible by more than 1 and themselves. Four, six, eight, and ten are composite numbers. For example, 24 is a composite number that is divisible by 1, 2, 3, 4, 6, 8, 12, and 24. *Content area:* Mathematics.

4. **(C)** Shakespeare, an English dramatist, wrote the play *Hamlet*. Homer, a Greek writer, wrote the epic *The Odyssey. Content area:* Humanities (literature).

5. **(B)** Portion and collection are antonyms, as are solid and powdery. *Content area:* English grammar, usage, and vocabulary.

6. **(D)** Living organisms are classified or grouped by scientific names. Members of the classification, Family, include Hominidae. Members of the classification, Genus, include *Homo. Content area:* Natural sciences (biology).

7. **(A)** Antietam and Shiloh were battles in the American Civil War. Bunker Hill and Valley Forge were battles in the American Revolutionary War. *Content area:* Social sciences (American history).

8. **(D)** A gaggle is a group of geese. A swarm is a group of bees. *Content area:* English grammar, usage, and vocabulary.

9. **(B)** Surnames are family names such as Jones, Walker, or Barlett. Pseudonyms are pen names or false names assumed by a writer. *Content area:* English grammar, usage, and vocabulary.

10. **(C)** One of the components or ingredients of bread is flour. One of the components or ingredients of an omelet is eggs. *Content area:* Commonplace information.

11. **(A)** Abide and abode are verbs. Abide is present tense and abode is past tense. The same is true for slink and slunk. Both are verbs with slink indicating present tense and slunk indicating past tense. *Content area:* English grammar, usage, and vocabulary.

12. **(B)** One part or component of an electrical system is wires. One part or component of a flower is petals. *Content area:* Commonplace information.

13. **(D)** The end result of running can be exhaustion, or running can cause exhaustion. An indicator of an infection is a fever, or an infection can cause a fever. *Content area:* Natural sciences (physiology).

14. **(C)** The musical term adagio means slow or a slow movement or piece of music. The musical term allegro means lively or a lively movement. The paired terms are synonyms. *Content area:* Humanities (music).

15. **(B)** One of the defining characteristics of the sun is that it gives off heat. One of the defining characteristics of a skunk is its distinctive odor. *Content area:* Commonplace information.

16. **(A)** A period of engagement usually precedes, or goes before, a marriage. A period or time of separation usually precedes a divorce. *Content area:* Social studies (behavioral sciences).

17. **(A)** John Donne, an English poet, wrote "Death Be Not Proud." Emily Dickinson, an American poet, wrote "Because I Could Not Stop For Death." *Content area:* Humanities (poetry).

18. **(D)** Paleozoic and Mesozoic are eras in geological time. Fishes, as life forms, appeared during the Paleozoic era; mammals, as life forms, appeared during the Mesozoic era. *Content area:* Natural sciences (earth science).

19. **(D)** Zeus was the king of the Greek gods. Jupiter was king of the Roman gods, or his Roman counterpart. Hades was the Greek god of the underworld; Pluto was his Roman counterpart. *Content area:* Humanities (mythology).

20. **(B)** Abstruse and rudimentary are antonyms, as are esoteric and elementary. Abstruse and esoteric are synonyms, as are rudimentary and elementary. *Content area:* English grammar, usage, and vocabulary.

21. **(A)** The northern lights are the common, everyday name for the Aurora Borealis. The southern lights are the common name for the Aurora Australis. The word aurora is defined as polar lights. Austral means southern, and boreal means northern. *Content area:* Natural sciences (earth science).

22. **(C)** The measurements are based on the metric system. One hectometer is 100 meters. One decameter is 10 meters. Hecto is a prefix meaning one hundred; deca is a prefix meaning ten. A meter is a length of 39.37 inches. *Content area:* Mathematics.

23. **(D)** The heart is responsible for the pumping or circulation of the blood. The lungs are responsible for the oxygenation of the blood. *Content area:* Natural sciences (biology).

24. **(B)** Piaget was a Swiss psychologist who formulated the stage theory of intellectual development. Kohlberg was an American psychologist who formulated the stages of moral development. *Content area:* Social sciences (psychology).

25. **(B)** The Declaration of Independence was authored by Thomas Jefferson. The Constitution of the United States was authored by many men, including James Madison. The Declaration of Independence and the Constitution of the United States are both documents that deal with the growth of democracy and establishment of the American nation. Both Jefferson and Madison were presidents of the United States. *Content area:* Social sciences (American history).

Answer Sheet
SAMPLE TEST TWO

Analogy

1 Ⓐ Ⓑ Ⓒ Ⓓ	10 Ⓐ Ⓑ Ⓒ Ⓓ	19 Ⓐ Ⓑ Ⓒ Ⓓ
2 Ⓐ Ⓑ Ⓒ Ⓓ	11 Ⓐ Ⓑ Ⓒ Ⓓ	20 Ⓐ Ⓑ Ⓒ Ⓓ
3 Ⓐ Ⓑ Ⓒ Ⓓ	12 Ⓐ Ⓑ Ⓒ Ⓓ	21 Ⓐ Ⓑ Ⓒ Ⓓ
4 Ⓐ Ⓑ Ⓒ Ⓓ	13 Ⓐ Ⓑ Ⓒ Ⓓ	22 Ⓐ Ⓑ Ⓒ Ⓓ
5 Ⓐ Ⓑ Ⓒ Ⓓ	14 Ⓐ Ⓑ Ⓒ Ⓓ	23 Ⓐ Ⓑ Ⓒ Ⓓ
6 Ⓐ Ⓑ Ⓒ Ⓓ	15 Ⓐ Ⓑ Ⓒ Ⓓ	24 Ⓐ Ⓑ Ⓒ Ⓓ
7 Ⓐ Ⓑ Ⓒ Ⓓ	16 Ⓐ Ⓑ Ⓒ Ⓓ	25 Ⓐ Ⓑ Ⓒ Ⓓ
8 Ⓐ Ⓑ Ⓒ Ⓓ	17 Ⓐ Ⓑ Ⓒ Ⓓ	
9 Ⓐ Ⓑ Ⓒ Ⓓ	18 Ⓐ Ⓑ Ⓒ Ⓓ	

Analogy Sample Test Two

Directions: For each of the questions, select the letter (A, B, C, or D) that makes the best match with the remaining analogous terms. Record your answers on the answer sheet on page 75.

1. FEMALE : OVARY :: _____ : _____

   (A) MALE : TESTIS
   (B) MALE : MEIOSIS
   (C) MALE : PENUMBRA
   (D) MALE : ORGAN

2. CAN : ABILITY :: MAY : _____

   (A) JUNE
   (B) CAPABILITY
   (C) PERMISSION
   (D) MOVEMENT

3. STALLION : HORSE :: ROOSTER : _____

   (A) SHAM
   (B) CHICKEN
   (C) HEN
   (D) SPUR

4. BUTTE : _____ :: CANYON : NARROW DEEP VALLEY

   (A) FAN-SHAPED AREA   CHALLENGE
   (B) BARREN LAND
   (C) ROUND-TOPPED HILL
   (D) MESA

5. ILLUSTRATION : FOR EXAMPLE :: ADDITIONAL ITEMS : _____

   (A) IN SUCH CASES
   (B) ACCORDINGLY
   (C) NEVERTHELESS
   (D) AS WELL AS

6. ALLEGORY : _____ :: COMEDY : *ALL'S WELL THAT ENDS WELL*

   (A) *PILGRIM'S PROGRESS*   CHALLENGE
   (B) *THE RIME OF THE ANCIENT MARINER*
   (C) *CHICAGO*
   (D) *GULLIVER'S TRAVELS*

7. 24/36 : 2/3 :: 12/64 : _____

   (A) 1/3
   (B) 3/16
   (C) 3/8
   (D) 6/32

8. PRINCIPLE : PRINCIPAL :: MEAT : _____

   (A) MEET
   (B) MET
   (C) MAT
   (D) MATE

9. PHARMACOLOGY : DRUGS :: CARDIOLOGY : _____

   (A) KIDNEYS
   (B) BODY MOVEMENT
   (C) HEART
   (D) DEATH

10. FARMER : HOE :: FISHERMAN : _____

   (A) BOAT
   (B) FISH
   (C) ROD
   (D) RIVER

11. _____ : MIXED ::
HOMOGENEOUS : UNIFORM

    (A) INGENIOUS
    (B) HETEROGENEOUS
    (C) MERETRICIOUS
    (D) LIGNEOUS

12. PERSONA NON GRATA : UNWELCOME
:: _____ : ACTING AS PARENT

    (A) ALFRESCO   [CHALLENGE]
    (B) ENFANT TERRIBLE
    (C) VENDETTA
    (D) IN LOCO PARENTIS

13. ISTANBUL : CONSTANTINOPLE :: HO
CHI MINH CITY : _____

    (A) BELIZE
    (B) CHAD
    (C) SAIGON
    (D) STALINGRAD

14. EDISON : PHONOGRAPH :: _____
: LIGHTNING ROD

    (A) FRANKLIN
    (B) WHITNEY
    (C) DIESEL
    (D) MARCONI

15. 2/5 : 40% :: _____ : 62.5%

    (A) 1/3
    (B) 5/8
    (C) 4/5
    (D) 1/6

16. LOUVRE : PARIS :: METROPOLITAN :
_____

    (A) ISTANBUL
    (B) BERLIN
    (C) NEW YORK
    (D) MADRID

17. KINGDOM : _____ :: SPECIES :
SAPIENS

    (A) CHORDATA
    (B) ORDER
    (C) GENUS
    (D) ANIMALIA

18. SPORES : AMPHIBIANS :: MODERN
MAMMALS : _____

    (A) FERNS
    (B) DINOSAURS
    (C) HUMANKIND
    (D) MARINE ALGAE

19. BOON : _____ :: BENEFACTION :
PRIVATION

    (A) BLESSING   [CHALLENGE]
    (B) DRAWBACK
    (C) LARGESS
    (D) DONATION

20. SECEDE : GEORGIA :: UNITE :
_____

    (A) ALABAMA
    (B) PENNSYLVANIA
    (C) ARIZONA
    (D) ARKANSAS

21. STADIUM : BLEACHERS :: CHURCH :
_____

    (A) PEWS
    (B) BENCHES
    (C) SEAT
    (D) CHAIRS

22. ENRAPTURE : _____ :: DISGUST:
REPEL

    (A) ENCASE
    (B) CLIMB
    (C) BEWITCH
    (D) DESCEND

23. SPRING : SUMMER :: 75 : _____

    (A) 12
    (B) 125
    (C) 50
    (D) 100

24. LAW : PEOPLE :: GOGGLES : _____

    (A) EYES
    (B) READING
    (C) PROTECTION
    (D) CONFINING

25. PERNICIOUS : HARMLESS ::
 PESTIFEROUS: _____

    (A) FATAL
            | CHALLENGE |
    (B) NOXIOUS
    (C) KIND
    (D) INIQUITOUS

Analogy Sample Test Two Answer Key

1. **(A)** The ovary is the egg-producing organ in the female of a species. The testis is the sperm-producing organ in the male of a species. *Content area:* Natural sciences (biology).

2. **(C)** The word *can* indicates an individual or group has the ability to do something. The word *may* indicates an individual or group is seeking permission to do something. *Content area:* English usage, grammar, and vocabulary.

3. **(B)** A stallion is a male horse capable of producing offspring. A rooster is a male chicken capable of producing offspring. *Content area:* Commonplace information.

4. **(C)** A butte is a round-topped hill. A canyon is a narrow deep valley. *Content area:* Natural sciences (earth science).

5. **(D)** In literature, transitional words are used to indicate or allude to the purpose of the presented details. "For example" is an expression that illustrates a general idea or impression. "As well as" is an expression that indicates that additional items are present. *Content area:* Humanities (literature).

6. **(A)** An allegory is a literary, dramatic, or pictorial piece in which abstract concepts, characters, events, or objects are presented in symbolic, concrete terms. *Pilgrim's Progress* is an example of an allegory. A comedy is a humorous literary, dramatic, or pictorial piece that has a happy ending. *All's Well That Ends Well* is an example of a comedy. *Content area:* Humanities (literature).

7. **(B)** The fraction 24/36 reduced to its lowest term is 2/3. The fraction 12/64 reduced to its lowest term is 3/16. This is accomplished by dividing both numbers by the largest number that divides evenly into both. Four is the largest number that evenly divides into 12/64. *Content area:* Mathematics.

8. **(A)** Principle and principal are homonyms or words that are pronounced the same but have different spellings and meaning. Meat and meet are also homonyms. *Content area:* English grammar, usage, and vocabulary.

9. **(C)** Pharmacology is the study of drugs and their interactions. Cardiology is the study of the heart. *Content area:* Natural sciences (biology/chemistry).

10. **(C)** A hoe is a hand-held tool used by a farmer. A rod or fishing rod is a hand-held tool used by a fisherman. *Content area:* Commonplace information.

11. **(B)** Heterogeneous and mixed are synonyms, as are homogeneous and uniform. *Content area:* Natural sciences (biology)

12. **(D)** Many foreign words and phrases have been incorporated in everyday English usage. *Persona non grata* is Latin and means an unwelcome person. *In loco parentis* is Latin and means in the place of a parent. *Content area:* English grammar, usage, and vocabulary.

13. **(C)** The names of many cities have changed over time. Constantinople is the previous name of the modern city of Istanbul, Turkey. Saigon is the previous name of the modern city of Ho Chi Minh City, Vietnam. *Content area:* Social studies (geography).

14. **(A)** Thomas Edison invented the phonograph. Benjamin Franklin invented the lightning rod. *Content area:* Social studies (history).

15. **(B)** Rational numbers may be presented as fractions or decimals. Two fifths and 40% are the same amount or quantity, as are 5/8 and 62.5%. To change a fraction to a percentage, divide the denominator, the bottom number, into the numerator, the upper number. *Content area:* Mathematics.

16. **(C)** The Louvre is in Paris. The Metropolitan is in New York. Both are world famous art museums. *Content area:* Humanities (art).

17. **(D)** Living organisms are classified according to taxonomy or taxonomic groups. Kingdom is the largest taxonomic unit. Animalia is an example found within this unit. The smallest taxonomic unit is the species of which *sapiens* is an example. *Content area:* Natural sciences (biology).

18. **(C)** According to geologic time, spores, as life forms, appeared prior to amphibians. Modern mammals, as life forms, appeared prior to mankind. *Content area:* Natural sciences (earth science).

19. **(B)** Boon and drawback are antonyms, as are benefaction and privation. Boon and benefaction are synonyms, as are drawback and privation. *Content area:* English grammar, usage, and vocabulary.

20. **(B)** During the Civil War, Georgia was one state to secede, or split away, from the Union. The state of Pennsylvania remained united with the Union. *Content area:* Social studies (history).

21. **(A)** Individuals sit in bleachers at a stadium. Bleachers are typically a part of a stadium. Individuals sit in pews in a church. Pews are typically a part of a church. *Content area:* English grammar, usage, and vocabulary.

22. **(C)** Enrapture and bewitch are synonyms, as are disgust and repel. *Content area:* English grammar, usage, and vocabulary.

23. **(D)** The season spring comes before summer, or summer follows spring. The number 75 comes before 100, the number 100 follows 75. Choice B is incorrect because 125 follows 100, not 75. *Content area:* Commonplace information.

24. **(A)** The purpose of the law is to protect people. The purpose of goggles is to protect the eyes. *Content area:* English grammar, usage, and vocabulary.

25. **(C)** Pernicious and harmless are antonyms, as are pestiferous and kind. Pernicious and pestiferous are synonyms, as are harmless and kind. *Content area:* English grammar, usage, and vocabulary.

Reading Comprehension

In Chapter 3 on verbal ability, you had an opportunity to formulate a plan for developing your vocabulary. To retain the words that you have learned, there is no substitute for practice. Reading on a daily basis and using new words in speech will be helpful. Keeping a notebook with unfamiliar words will allow you to check meanings later so that you can add words to your daily speech. If you practice analyzing words now, your efforts will pay off when you take tests, as well as in daily work life.

Once again, as in the chapter on test-taking strategies, actual nursing school entrance exams may or may not have the specific topics that are provided in this chapter. Practice with actual nursing school entrance exam topics comes later in this text. This chapter will enhance your test-taking skills through practice with reading short passages, identifying the major theme of each passage, recalling specific facts, making inferences about the story in each passage, and deciphering any new vocabulary. These skills will be applied when you take the nursing school entrance exam. Though vocabulary is important to reading comprehension, it also involves identification of themes within the passages read.

Vocabulary building could be said to be a relatively narrow skill when compared to reading comprehension. Even though you may understand the individual words in a passage that you read, you may not be able to grasp the main themes of the passage successfully. In order to develop this ability to identify main themes, practice is necessary. You must practice the skill of learning vocabulary words and then expand this knowledge into the broader skill of identifying main themes.

To better understand this need to develop two sets of skills, consider the nearsighted person who can examine every aspect of a single tree but cannot recognize the entire forest because poor distance vision renders the forest as a dull blur. This individual is tuned in to the details but cannot focus on the big picture. Even though you may be able to successfully read and understand individual sentences, you need to expand this skill into an ability to read a passage, paragraph, or set of paragraphs and to make overall sense of the messages conveyed.

This chapter offers excellent practice for what will come later, should you enter nursing school. Nursing requires a fine-tuned skill known as critical thinking. It involves the ability to take sets of facts, combine these with all possible related facts, and form correct assumptions upon which to act. Nursing decision making rests on a foundation of expertise in critical thinking. Critical thinking, in turn, is based upon the ability to analyze a situation. And an excellent way to hone your analysis skills is to practice analyzing what you read and hear.

In the next section, we will examine some passages of text for main themes. The first selection is about osteoporosis. You will be asked to identify main themes and to respond to questions about the main themes. Then, you will be given an exercise that will show you how to select new words and incorporate them into your daily speech. At first, this will seem tedious but, with practice, it will become more automatic.

Introduction to Practice at Reading Comprehension

Test items involving reading comprehension appear to be complex but are often among the simplest types to sort out and answer. Indeed, the techniques used to respond to reading comprehension questions often involve nothing more than sorting out the information contained in a paragraph. Typically, reading comprehension questions consist of a reading selection followed by a series of questions designed to discover whether the test taker really understood what was said in the paragraph.

For example, the following paragraph contains a great deal of information, and the two questions that follow it ask the test taker to respond to small bits of data. Notice that the questions use words different from those found in the paragraph, in order to ensure that the test taker is not parroting information about which understanding was weak.

Experts feel that there has been an alarming increase in osteoporosis. This disease is also known as "brittle bone disease." Osteoporosis has long been linked to calcium and vitamin D intake. There is the persistent notion that osteoporosis is more prevalent in those with a lifetime pattern of insufficient calcium intake. However, as with many such diseases, low calcium intake is not sufficient, in the absence of other factors, to produce this disease. Osteoporosis is prevalent in women past the age of menopause. Often, in women diagnosed with osteoporosis, there is a strong family history of brittle bone disease. Osteoporosis may result in stooped posture in old age. The disease may not become apparent until the elderly female, or in some cases the elderly male, suffers an actual fracture. Diagnostic tests include a noninvasive technique that measures bone density and that is similar to x-ray procedures. There is controversy regarding the safety of hormone replacement therapy. Since osteoporosis tends to occur in women who are postmenopausal, it is logical to assume that hormone substitution would be effective in preventing the disease in those at high risk. However, there is substantial evidence that long-term hormone replacement therapy may place women at risk for other, sometimes fatal, disease processes. Therefore, this preventive treatment needs to be carefully considered on an individual basis.

Question 1

What would be the best advice to give your neighbor who has just heard a news report that osteoporosis is on the rise?

(A) You should be fine as long as you have your annual checkups.
(B) It does not hit until old age, and since you are only 40, there is no need to worry yet.
(C) Taking sufficient calcium with vitamin D is one way in which you might help yourself.
(D) Physicians are the appropriate persons to give advice, and others are not legally allowed to do so.

COMMENTS:

The correct response is C. Notice that the paragraph does not explicitly state that taking calcium is considered a possible preventive measure. The reader must infer this. The phrases "insufficient calcium intake" and "lifetime pattern" are key phrases. They should lead you to realize that a lifetime pattern of sufficient calcium intake won't hurt and could possibly help. Indeed, some test takers underline key passages in the paragraph, in order to sort out useful from unhelpful information within the paragraph.

In the case of this sample, choice D was not addressed in the paragraph at all and seems like a too-convenient pat answer.

You also have doubts about choice A: the one that implies that having routine annual checkups will lead to detection of osteoporosis. You decide that your neighbor's interests would not be served by choosing this response.

That leaves two choices. Choice B addresses the old age issue and choice C deals with calcium intake. At this point, you should return to the reading selection and locate the part that discusses old age and underline or highlight it. You should do the same with the calcium section. You then review this material to determine exactly what the paragraph says. In this case, the paragraph refers to heredity, age, and calcium intake as associated with osteoporosis. But you finally decide, based on nothing more than your impression that the paragraph information seems to lead more logically to choice C, concerning calcium. Also, you don't favor choice B because it sounds like an absolute statement—one of those pesky black-and-white phrases that are seldom correct in the realm of human function. Choice B indicates that one should postpone worrying. The implication is that osteoporosis would *never* occur before one is 60 years old or so. Absolute statements or implications such as this are seldom correct.

But what sorts of information would you look for if this were a particularly long and complex paragraph and if the question being asked was especially difficult? To become adept and relatively fearless at handling such paragraphs, you must practice reading with absolute confidence and sorting through information. Techniques for training yourself to be able to handle more complex material are covered in the next section on reading practice patterns.

But, before moving on to develop your ability to recall and understand themes, return to the paragraph on osteoporosis and select some words for which you do not know the definitions. To illustrate how to practice making these new word patterns part of your permanent vocabulary, let us use the word *prevalent* from the osteoporosis section, as well as the word phrases *noninvasive technique* and *persistent notion*. First, before you go to the dictionary, try to find any prefixes that help to decipher the word. You note that *non* and *invasive* are used, and you know that non means not and that invasive means a sort of threat to enter into something or somewhere. When you look up *noninvasive*, you notice that you were right on target. Next, imagine yourself later in the day and on the next day, trying to insert some of the words and phrases into your speech. You may even want to tell your family and coworkers what you're up to so that they don't look at you strangely. Friends, coworkers, and family may make a bit of fun at first, but, in the long run, they will no doubt respect your efforts to expand your word mastery and analysis skills.

Reading Practice Patterns

For those individuals who read slowly or who have difficulty in pulling out the facts once you have read something, you should practice reading anything and everything.

When you are armed with a formidable selection of things to enlighten, inform, and increase your ability to decipher complex paragraphs or short passages, find your space to put your plan in action. In the real test situation, you will be required to sit in your seat and concentrate on text passages for many long minutes, or even hours. Put a clipboard, paper, and writing implement close at hand.

You must practice concentrating in the absence of televison, radio, or other familiar background noises. Record the sounds of someone chewing gum or pencils falling off a table; you may even want to throw in some sneezes or throat clearing. Professional golfers, when they are young and learning to concentrate, often ask friends or family to whistle, shout, or throw things into their field of vision as they are about to swing at the ball. The novice golfer actually practices concentrating in the face of distraction. You should do the same.

As you practice reading, keep in mind that, on a test, knowledge of the subject matter is not enough. You need the sort of stamina that you will develop through practice. Developing this type of concentration will enable you to focus on the matter at hand and to do your best in any testing situation.

In the case of the person studying to do well on a nursing entrance test, it is imperative that the individual get used to silent rooms and be able to withstand distractions in order to concentrate on reading. You need to practice comprehending all types of reading material. Repetitive practice, whether you are doing private reading or taking the practice examinations at the end of this book, will also increase your ability to read the passage quickly and comprehend it completely. You will get done with the test in timely fashion and should feel good about the test as you leave.

As the weeks of practice go on, try to select more difficult material from the library. In addition to reading for whole-paragraph or whole-passage comprehension in general, be sure to write down any new or unfamiliar words for vocabulary enhancement and analysis.

In relation to the actual techniques useful in reading for comprehension, you will now use the clipboard. In order to effectively answer questions following moderately or severely complex paragraphs, you need to go through a series of steps. The first step is an initial reading, which will tell you that the paragraph is complicated. At this time, skim the material; don't try to examine each little detail.

Next, in a few sentences, write a summary of the main ideas. Do not look back at the paragraph. When you have jotted down your summary, look back at the selection and see if you missed anything. Do nothing more than quickly reading and summarizing the passage during your first few days of practice.

With repetition, you will have started to comprehend what is needed in each paragraph by reading it through once for general understanding. This ability will be invaluable at test time. You will be able to read with confidence and know that you have grasped the essentials.

Some people recommend that you underline key words or phrases instead of summarizing the selection following the initial reading. It is my experience that this can be helpful if not carried to extremes.

TIP

For practice at theme identification, try the sample theme paragraphs at the end of this chapter.

Question Scanning

In the actual test situation, after your initial reading, you should scan each question that follows the paragraph and then reread each choice to determine whether they all seem reasonable to you.

Returning to our sample situation concerning osteoporosis, recall that the paragraph had several main themes. Close your eyes at this point and see if you can recall some. Then go on to scan the following listing:

1. Osteoporosis is brittle bone disease.
2. Osteoporosis is associated with bone fractures and disfiguring spinal curvatures in older age groups.
3. Osteoporosis strikes more women than men.
4. There are a couple of tests available to tell whether one is at risk.
5. Calcium deficiency may be involved, so it might be a good idea to take sufficient calcium throughout life.
6. In women, postmenopause is the key time for osteoporosis development. Therefore, some care providers recommend hormone replacement despite its risks.

You should have been able to identify at least half of these key elements. Any others would have been retrievable, but were not the first to spring into your mind.

After you have identified the key paragraph elements, it is time to scan responses. Consider the following sets of response choices based on the osteoporosis paragraph.

Question 2

Your neighbor states that the calcium idea is a good one and that she will try it. However, she is still worried, since her aunt was hospitalized with a fractured hip last year and subsequently died of complications of prolonged bedrest. Your neighbor fears that this will happen to her someday. What is your best response?

(A) "There are simple mechanical and radiologic tests that can diagnose this disease. Why don't you call the local clinics and find out who is administering these tests these days?"

(B) "Your posture seems really straight. You'll know if you have the disease because you'll start to look a little bit stooped when you stand up. I doubt that you have it, though. I don't see any bend at all."

(C) "Treatments are getting better all the time. By the time you're as old as your aunt, they'll have something to fix it, I suspect. So you need to not worry so much. Do you usually worry about things a lot?"

(D) "You should take hormones as soon as your doctor permits it. This will delay the full effects of menopause and most cases of osteoporosis occur after menopause."

COMMENTS:

Scan the possible responses in light of the highlights you have saved in your mind or on paper. You should also place yourself in the situation and try to see which choices feel the most comfortable.

Choice A deals with having your neighbor seek some testing. This response feels fairly comfortable and is in line with one of the themes of the paragraph (checklist item 4) so you don't rule it out. You need to keep in mind that you like choice A fairly well.

Choice B deals with reassuring your neighbor that she looks fine to you and is therefore probably fine. This response makes you really uncomfortable. You have been visualizing a neighbor you really like, and you can see what it would mean to her if you were wrong. You discard choice B.

Choice C is another general reassurance response and you think that it is not as sound as choice A. You discard it.

Choice D seems quite logical and fits many of the facts you remember from the paragraph. The problem is that you recall something about hormones being somewhat controversial. You decide that your neighbor needs some reassurance and sound advice, and she may best get really sound advice through testing by professionals. You feel quite justified in sticking with choice A, which happens to be the correct answer.

Let's look at another reading comprehension exercise. Read the following paragraphs and respond to the question that follows.

Simulations are replications linked to some facet of phenomena. They exist operationally as real or symbolic and are engineered to communicate relevant data that can be utilized in creating and improving that which has been developed. The use of such a model is today very applicable to the social sciences.

Information is produced that impacts processes. True understanding of this fact is evident in analyzing simulation techniques with collected data. Simulation is a consistent evaluative tool, in that it represents constant justification of the obtained data along with in-the-moment content and context of the creative processes. Simulation, especially in nursing, models both expected and unexpected behavior. For example, when used in the context of nursing, simulation is interchangeable with interviewing, experimenting or trialing, and/or observation, followed with secondary analyses to the contrary of the original. In nursing, simulation allows for learning by way of expected error without realistic consequences as a result of the learning. Thus, simulation learning expectations are not in competition with traditional real-life expectations, which are used to critique and even improve the data produced from the simulation.

Nursing simulation procedures or skills primarily centers on the pre-clinical goals being accomplished, along with those that are evident and applicable in the moment, with the scope of understanding priority during the process of learning. Therefore, inclusive phenomena have an affect on initial phenomena created for investigation. New data are now available to determine if they co-exist, as emerged from the combination of previous simulation expectations and discovered knowledge.

Simulation is pliable in that much can be explored given numerous processes. Simulation is amendable to variety secondary to discovery. Computer simulation lends itself to creative variations with immediate discovery of results and implications. Numerous factors can be manipulated, i.e., numbers, subjects, and results to name a few. Choice selections are programmable at the manipulator's whim. Unexpected results can be determined and changed within a blink of an eye. A host of theories of choice behavior are timely predicted. These changed theories can be mathematical or logistical terms that are perhaps tested against actual data as correlated with choices of live participants.

When distinguishing between computer simulation and non-computer simulation, the determining factor relates to one being designed and the other being controlled by a specific theory. The computer simulation is manipulated with diverse choices, creating various behaviors. The unexpected results with this method can be quite surprising and beneficial to the investigator. The non-computer simulation is patterned after the selected theory where results are pretty much guaranteed based on predetermined factors; that is, behavior is predictable. The investigator continues to work at achieving results that may be useful for computer simulation.

Hence, simulation, whether in combination with computer or not, may result in the futility of the investigator's research knowledge integrated with theoretical knowledge that leads to phenomenal data in predicting behavior useful in teaching and learning.

This passage is lengthy. It is important to apply the reading skills learned thus far to understand the two sides of the issue. The point of view is diverse throughout the passage. There is the subtle implication that computer simulation allows the researcher to vary the data for immediate discovery and that non-computer simulation is a challenging secondary to implicit-driven behavior.

Read the passage in its entirety; then scan the paragraphs, highlighting a few key points:

1. Simulations are replications linked to some facet of phenomena
2. Real or symbolic
3. Engineered to communicate relevant data that can be utilized in creating and improving that which has been developed
4. A consistent evaluative tool
5. In nursing, models both expected and unexpected behavior
6. Inclusive phenomena affect initial phenomena created for investigation
7. Determining factor relates to one being designed and the other being controlled by a specific theory

Before advancing to the question, try visualizing yourself being involved in both a nursing computer-simulation and a nursing non-computer situation to perhaps gain an appreciation of the diversity of each type.

Now you are ready to go on. Try your hand at the following routine question.

Question 3

Which of the following statements about simulation is correct?

(A) Simulation is constant.
(B) Simulation could never be real.
(C) There is only one type of theory used with simulation.
(D) Simulation communicates relevant data that can be utilized in improving that which has been developed.

COMMENTS:

If you have made an effective list of facts from the passage, and if you have visualized the situation, answering this question will be simple. Simulation communicates relevant data that can be utilized in improving that which has been developed (choice D).

In synopsizing the passage, you need to be able to put your finger on key points. During a test, whenever you encounter a complex passage involving words that are not instantly familiar, assume that the questions will involve at least one of these words. You may even need to visualize yourself involved in the activities suggested by these words. Making your own simplified listings will also help. If you are unable to bring paper into the actual test, write listings on the test booklet. If you are unable to do that, then try to visualize your listings.

The next example will definitely illustrate the complex type of passage. Again, as you read the paragraphs in the passage, try to picture the situation and what all those new and unfamiliar terms are doing at any one time. Then make a short list from memory, associating each new term with what it means, but do not spend a lot of time looking back at the paragraphs. Use your memory instead.

If you are in a test situation and time is running short, read through the questions at the end of the selection before you do any other reading. Then read the selection, and make your own list of what *those* terms mean.

An example of a complex passage follows. After reading this selection, answer the two reading comprehension questions.

Every two to seven years a weather phenomenon known as El Niño appears. For the year during which its effects last, it is said to have a global influence, even though it is mainly a Pacific Ocean phenomenon. El Niño is interesting to American meteorologists for its effects along the seacoasts and in the flat lands of the midwest in the United States. In an El Niño year, beaches along the west coast of South America are balmy even in winter. South American fisheries have larger harvests, while North American marine creatures have very diminished food supplies. Marine life may even die off in the northern hemisphere. There are fewer tornadoes and hurricanes in North America. The Asian monsoons are lighter, and Australia may go through a period of drought.

Why is this? Normally trade winds blow across the Pacific from east to west (from the Americas toward Asia). These trade winds carry the surface ocean water with them. They dump a great deal of moisture in Asia. Along the eastern Pacific, the trade winds cause cool, deep ocean water to rise to the surface to replace that which is missing (the water that traveled to the west with the trade winds). The cooler water along the eastern Pacific, which touches the American states of California, Oregon, and Washington, comes to the surface. Plankton and other small creatures feed well. This maintains the food supply for larger fish and marine mammals in the northern hemisphere. Meanwhile, in the western Pacific, the monsoon rains pour down, and Australia and New Zealand can count on normal amounts of moisture.

During an El Niño year, the trade winds are light and the water doesn't travel to the west. The surface water all over the Pacific is warm. Monsoons fall off, and Australia goes dry. There is no rise to the surface of cool, deeper water along the California coast. Plankton levels fall.

Question 4

Which of the following can be said about El Niño?

(A) El Niño is a dangerous phenomenon, causing a tremendous increase in the number of tornadoes in the United States. Scientists should work to understand and, perhaps, eliminate it.

(B) El Niño disrupts the usual weather patterns all over the globe.

(C) El Niño causes flooding in Australia.

(D) El Niño usually lasts for about seven years.

COMMENTS:

Having read the passage, close your eyes and picture what it said. If you are confused, realize that this is an extremely complex type of paragraph for a nonmeteorologist. Read it again while picturing which way the wind blows and which way the water goes (east, west; up, down). You may want to draw two small diagrams that fit the facts of the paragraph. Draw Asia and Australia on the left and the Americas on the right in both diagrams. Label one picture "El Niño Year" and the other "Not an El Niño Year."

On the ordinary (Not an El Niño Year) map, draw little trade wind symbols showing them blowing from America toward Asia. Make a note that water is traveling toward Asia with the trade winds. Draw little typhoons happening over Asia. Show Australia having rain and being green. On the right side of your diagram, show deep water coming up to the surface along California and little fish and yummy green plankton proliferating on the surface. Fishing and climate are as usual in South America, and tornadoes and hurricanes are doing their usual thing in North America. Look back at the paragraph and note that this situation prevails for from one to six years.

On the El Niño map show that the El Niño situation prevails for about one year. Show no trade winds (an exaggeration, but you do not care). Show dryness over Australia (remember that surface ocean water did not have a chance to travel all the way to the west with the trade winds) and no little monsoons over Asia. Show a drop in normal levels of hurricanes and tornadoes over North America. Show unhappy fish along the coast of California, since the deep water never came to the surface and never brought up the smaller fish and green plankton to eat. Show South American beaches being balmy in winter.

Now you are ready to respond to the previous question. It becomes quite simple because you can immediately rule out choices A, C, and D. These responses do not match your diagrams. During El Niño, there is no dangerous increase in the number of tornadoes in the United States so choice A does not fit. You note that during El Niño flooding in Australia does not happen but that dryness does. Goodbye to choice C. You also note that El Niño does not last seven years so there goes choice D.

Question 5

What can be inferred about the connection between trade winds and El Niño?

(A) Trade winds normally blow from the western United States to Asia. Therefore, between El Niño years, there are more monsoons.

(B) There is no connection between trade winds and El Niño.

(C) After trade winds complete their trans-Pacific journey, they continue across the Atlantic. That is why this is said to be a global phenomenon.

(D) During El Niño times, fish kills are more heavy throughout Asia and Australia because of the increase in winds and the fall-off in ocean food supplies such as plankton.

COMMENTS:

You should note immediately that choice A fits the facts. You may not even look farther, but, if you do, you will note that none of the other statements match the situations you sketched in your diagrams.

Putting It All Together

Using the test samples in this book and your own private reading selections, you can develop speed and skill with reading, recalling, and sketching the main themes found in reading passages. Find difficult readings on topics you know almost nothing about. Weekly news magazines often have sections dealing with the economy or with politicians taking different sides of complicated issues. Find these difficult passages and practice making short listings or diagrams. Then check back to see if your sketches or lists were correct. In addition to improving speed and comprehension, regularly pursuing these exercises will also help you search reading selections automatically for the main ideas so that you can save much of your mental energy for other things. And it will also build your confidence in yourself.

The reading comprehension questions in the practice tests at the end of this book contain time indicators so that you can test yourself to see if you are able to select main themes accurately and without wasting too much time. To read a lengthy passage and respond, you are given two and a half minutes per test question, or item; however, the last few test items call for you to be really speedy, allowing only one and a half minutes per item. These indicators will allow you to gauge your speed against other typical college students taking standardized, timed tests.

But what if you have only a very short time to prepare for the test? What if you have only days instead of the weeks or months that would enable you to practice thoroughly? The next section will advise the person in a hurry.

Problems of Limited Time

For those with just a few days or a week to prepare for the test, clear the decks. If you have a job, discuss with your boss the need to be away. If you have a family, clear some days away from intensive family responsibilities.

Then, find a quiet place. Read the chapters of this book and simply take as many of the tests as time will allow. You may not emerge as the perfect test taker, but you will have developed several talents. Not only will you be very familiar with the multiple-choice format, but also you will have had a chance to practice elimination and narrowing techniques with a variety of test items. In addition, you will have forced yourself to concentrate for long periods of time.

It is your responsibility to develop a quiet place and quiet times during which there will be no interruptions. Developing these times away from other commitments is not a selfish act on your part. You are thinking of a nursing career, and this will, in the long run, be something that will benefit you and your family or other associates. So give it all you've got and back away from other commitments. Ensure that the children and other responsibilities are taken care of, and use the time you have to prepare for your first step toward a nursing career.

Answer Sheet
SAMPLE TEST

Reading Comprehension

1 Ⓐ Ⓑ Ⓒ Ⓓ

2 Ⓐ Ⓑ Ⓒ Ⓓ

3 Ⓐ Ⓑ Ⓒ Ⓓ

4 Ⓐ Ⓑ Ⓒ Ⓓ

5 Ⓐ Ⓑ Ⓒ Ⓓ

6 Ⓐ Ⓑ Ⓒ Ⓓ

7 Ⓐ Ⓑ Ⓒ Ⓓ

8 Ⓐ Ⓑ Ⓒ Ⓓ

9 Ⓐ Ⓑ Ⓒ Ⓓ

10 Ⓐ Ⓑ Ⓒ Ⓓ

11 Ⓐ Ⓑ Ⓒ Ⓓ

12 Ⓐ Ⓑ Ⓒ Ⓓ

13 Ⓐ Ⓑ Ⓒ Ⓓ

14 Ⓐ Ⓑ Ⓒ Ⓓ

15 Ⓐ Ⓑ Ⓒ Ⓓ

Reading Comprehension Sample Test

Directions: For each of the questions, select the letter (A, B, C, or D) that best answers the question. Record your answers on the answer sheet on page 95.

Read the following passage and then answer the questions that follow.

Mineralogy is the study and science of minerals. Minerals consist of solid or liquid material having chemical and physical properties that are found in the earth. In comparison to minerals, rocks are very different. People have been interested in minerals for centuries. There are approximately 3000 known minerals. There are numerous minerals that are often transparent with nice colors or forms. The actual design and makeup of a particular mineral whether it becomes known as a precious stone or not is considered precious.

The formation: There are three developing processes: the magmatic developing process, the sedimentary developing process, and the metamorphic developing process. The magma is material associated with volcanoes and the lava. It is a liquid in the earth with a temperature of 1300 degrees. Once magma reaches the surface of the earth, it becomes colder and crystallizes. One of the last phases is the hydrothermal phase. In this phase some gases leave the magma flowing to the top. The gases form rooms in the rocks, which later are filled with magma. At this phase, quartz (rock crystal, amethyst) is initiated in its formation. Quartz is often associated with closed rooms of rock that are labeled as geodes. Quartz normally grows in cracks of rock. Environmental elements, such as water and wind can cause minerals to be deposited at the bottom of a liquid, resulting in a consolidation. This distinct process, linked with high temperatures allows for the development of new chemical creations. For example, with a great deal of force, frost can be changed, resulting highly dynamically. The mixture of water and oxygen while dispensed in the air permeates the development of new minerals, such as sedimentary. The metamorphic presents itself even more forcefully; thereby, allowing magma to flow in-between the rocks where minerals previously exist. It is the magma at this point that changes minerals.

Chemical and physical properties: Minerals are unique in that each is known for its specific chemical and physical properties, developing structures that will forever be recognized individually. The majority of minerals fall into categories of molecules or ions. There are nine classes:

1. Elements (diamond, gold, silver)
2. Sulfides, selenides, tellurides, arsenides, antimonides, and bismutides (pyrite)
3. Halides (fluorite, rock salt)
4. Oxides and hydroxides (corundum, quartz)
5. Nitrates, carbonates, and borates (calcite, malachite)
6. Sulfates, chromates, molybdates, and tungstenates (alabaster)

7. Phosphates, arsenates, and vanadates (turkis)
8. Silicates (feldspar, topaz)
9. Organic connections (amber)

A good number of minerals form crystals (cubical, monoclinical, triclinical, hexagonal, trigonal, tetragonal, rhombical). Rock salt for example crystallizes in the cubical form. Quartz and corundum (ruby, sapphire) crystallize in the trigonal system. During the formation phase, it is expected that the material will develop in its standard form, but if this does not occur as usual, the crystal is considered imperfect. This imperfect development can occur if the room is too small during the crystal formation phase or if other imperfect materials are utilized. This is important considering that crystals are hardly ever found to be perfect. There is an imperfectness associated with the perimeter and the height; they are never the same. Other properties known are the density, the hardness (the hardness is capable of breaking into a mineral). The Mohs' hardness scale measures from 1 to 10 and is used to accomplish accuracy. If a mineral has a hardness of 1, this translates into the mineral being sensitive enough to be scratched by a fingernail. On the opposite end of appreciating this fact is the diamond with a hardness of 10 would not be affected if an attempt was made to scratch it with a knife. Thus, a mineral with a higher hardness can scratch a mineral with a lower hardness. Minerals can be of a colorless nature; for example, diamond.

1. Based on the discussion of the hardness of minerals in the passage, which of the following minerals would you select as being the hardest?

   (A) Quartz
   (B) Topaz
   (C) Biotite
   (D) Diamond

2. Which of the following correctly describes minerals?

   (A) Minerals are classified by their formation.
   (B) Minerals are classified by their chemical composition and physical properties.
   (C) Minerals are mineraloids.
   (D) Minerals contain a standard structure.

3. If a metamorphic rock is combined with a sedimentary rock, what type of rock would it form?

   (A) Ancient
   (B) Metamorphic
   (C) Sedimentary
   (D) Granite

Read the following paragraphs about the passage of time and then answer the following questions that follow.

There is much written about time and its existence. The Greeks referred time to Chronos and Kairos. Chronos reflects chronological time, while Kairos is viewed more as a moment in time (no specific attachment of time); situations occur whenever decided by an individual. Life happens in the moment. One important developed factor over time dealt with the relationship of man and time, focusing on how man measured time. First, time was measured by analyzing cycles; for example, measuring time by movements of the moon and the sun. Later, these cycles were studied looking at the effects of time on nature, effects on seasons.

In the modern world, time is reflected in terms of hours, minutes, and seconds. As time became a factor in people's lives, the conscience of time attached control into the processes of existing and living. Humans live relating time to three perspectives: physics, metaphysics, and ethics. Physically, time is measured. Metaphysics correlates with feelings. Ethics involves linking time with actual living; that is, what are people doing with their time.

The invention of the clock increased the awareness of the passing of time. Beyond this fact, humans began to attach variable living situations to time, factoring time into actions of living and involvement with others; therefore, time is now correlated with feeling. For example, five minutes in a classroom is longer than fifteen minutes listening to an infamous physicist with a girl-friend or boyfriend. Ethically, time relates to the heart. Time is proportionate to the act of living. Time relates to the quality of living. Humans attach time with feeling, and this equates to measuring time.

It is challenging to develop strategies to manage personal time. Humans have to evaluate what they value and connect the value(s) to time, followed by time management. There are twenty-four hours in each day for each person. Some are able to accomplish numerous personal goals without a hitch: build new relationships, have fun, and care for self, work, and study. There are others who struggle to control their time. The key relates to making choices, organizing personal values, and creating strategies to achieve what's important relating to time.

4. The "feeling" in paragraph three is best defined as

   (A) the importance of time attached to the act of living.
   (B) sincere knowledge and love.
   (C) a yearning to be loved.
   (D) time is of essence.

5. What is the overall theme of the paragraphs?

   (A) Visions of living
   (B) Organizing one's life
   (C) The intervention of the clock
   (D) The relationship of man and time

6. Which statement is accurate about the three perspectives (*physics*, *metaphysics*, and *ethics*) of living?

    (A) Humans base living on love, family, and success.
    (B) Humans live by listening, learning, and leading.
    (C) Humans live relating time to physical, feeling, and living aspects.
    (D) Humans live relating time to working physically, consciousness, and living.

7. The initial discussion of "Greek historians" is primarily to

    (A) illustrate man and time as an issue since the beginning of time.
    (B) give credit where credit is due.
    (C) depict a setting for the discussion of time.
    (D) introduce another viewpoint.

8. The example in paragraph three is used to illustrate

    (A) time spent in a classroom is too short.
    (B) time listening to a physicist lecture is valuable.
    (C) time correlates with feeling, others, and quality.
    (D) time is scarce and more is needed in living.

Read the following paragraph about health and safety and then answer the questions that follow. You will be asked to state the main theme of the paragraph.

The "Fen/Phen" scare of 1997 revolved around the use of mood-altering medications for weight control. In some cases, use of these drugs resulted in heart valve damage, with resultant permanent disability and untimely death. This latest and most dramatic case of health risk from mood-altering substances has involved the concurrent use of fenfluramine and phentermine. Fenfluramine boosts levels of serotonin, a positive mood substance, and dopamine. Although fenfluramine works, it may make the person drowsy. So, to counteract this effect, phentermine, an amphetamine mimic that raises metabolism and alertness, was added. Taken together, these two drugs helped individuals to lose weight.

9. What is the main theme of the paragraph?

    (A) The Fen/Phen scare was just that—a scare, without any basis in fact.
    (B) Fen/Phen is safe and effective for weight loss when taken as directed.
    (C) Fen/Phen does not work.
    (D) Fen/Phen works but is dangerous.

10. Which statement is accurate according to the Fen/Phen paragraph?

    (A) Fenfluramine and phentermine both produce drowsiness.
    (B) Fenfluramine is associated with drowsiness; phentermine, with alertness.
    (C) Fenfluramine and phentermine both are associated with increased alertness.
    (D) Fenfluramine is associated with alertness; phentermine, with drowsiness.

Timed Reading and Response

The following paragraph is intended to rate your ability to read at a speed consistent with that of other nursing students while comprehending what you have read. Should you time yourself and determine that you read too slowly, you may want to practice. Reading too slowly or with too little comprehension could handicap you as you begin to read textbooks and nursing articles in preparation for classes.

Some nursing school entrance exams have timed-reading exercises and others do not. However, if you take the timed-reading exercise that follows and are slow to complete it, you may perhaps be in danger on an actual timed section of a nursing school entrance exam. There may be an additional problem involved with timed reading. If English is your second language and you find that you are not doing well on timed-reading segments as you practice with this book, be sure to contact your local university or college to ask for assistance. Often, there are even college clubs formed to assist and support those who learned their basic English-language skills in other countries.

Use an egg timer or have someone time you as you read. Select a pen or pencil so that you will be able to mark the point in the passage at which you stop reading. When you are ready to begin, have your timer set for one minute. Then begin to time and to read. When you have read for one minute, make a mark next to the line at which you stopped reading. You will later count down the number of lines of text you read in one minute. This will be your reading rate. The rate will be explained in the answer key.

Now set the timer for seven minutes. Continue reading until you have completed the entire passage. Respond to the questions attached to the passage. Do not try to look back at the associated paragraph at too great a length because this will waste time. During the seven-minute period, respond to the first question and go on reading and answering questions until time runs out. Scoring instructions and interpretation are explained in the answer key.

> **Directions:** Set the timer for one minute and mark your place at the end of one minute. After you have made your one-minute mark, set the timer for seven minutes and continue to read and answer questions until the seven minutes is up.

Section I

The great nursing leader, Florence Nightingale came from a privileged background. In England, at the time she was born, ladies of her class were expected to learn the arts and how to manage a household. They were raised with the expectation that they would marry an equally privileged individual and settle into a life of almost constant social activity and domestic management. Florence Nightingale chose to do otherwise. Among other unusual youthful activities, she spent part of her time touring Europe and the Middle East. She spent time at a renowned German training school for health care workers and eventually began inviting intellectuals and artists of the day to visit with her in her Paris salon. Apparently, her parents and her sister went along with this unusual activity, expressing concern only when she chose nursing as a vocation.

From a young age, Florence demonstrated a love of learning and an ability to think independently. She also enjoyed showing her disregard of what others might think. For example, she had a pet owl at a time when this was an unusual pet. One can imagine that she enjoyed surprising houseguests by displaying the owl. She even had her picture painted with the creature in hand.

Florence was raised in the countryside in elegant surroundings: a large house and spacious lawns, by current standards. As a young student, she was able to quickly master subjects from books and home lessons, such as the languages and music practice popular for young ladies of the age. But she went beyond these lessons to master other subjects and to engage in discussions, weighing the meaning of some of the knowledge acquired and perfecting her skills at drawing others out and engaging in peaceful debate.

During this childhood and teenage period, it is probable that she was quite successful at mastering some of the skills involved with being a good hostess. She would later be able to attract people to her dwelling in Paris for discussions and the sharing of ideas. This ability to attract the rich and powerful meant that she provided physical comfort when such guests would drop by. She must also have been able to provide stimulation through discussion or discussion leading.

It is no doubt from some of Florence Nightingale's early childhood experience that she derived her skills at melding the ideas of others into a new way of acting. In addition, practice in her childhood and early adult years with handling unconventional ideas and at softening the hard edges of debate allowed her to spread her ideas successfully as she dealt later with the powerful male and female figures of the time. That is, had she been strictly cold and authoritarian when approaching the important gate keepers of her age, or had she given in to a tendency to form grudges, she might have been correct in principle, but she would have been blocked at achieving change.

It is probable that Florence Nightingale was equally adept as an innovator and as a persuader. She was able to take ideas, gain access to proving grounds, or the field, test her ideas for accuracy, and then sell these ideas to those in positions of power. Another great inventor of new ideas, Thomas Edison, was also thrust into certain situations as a young person: those of experimenting with new ideas (the inventor side of his personality) and in selling ideas to others (his salesman side). Perhaps the same can be said of Florence Nightingale.

11. Which is an accurate synopsis (summary) of section I?

   (A) Florence Nightingale was rich but became poor.
   (B) Florence Nightingale chose to forsake her life of wealth and privilege to pursue a stronger interest.
   (C) Florence Nightingale spent part of her youth touring Europe and the Middle East.
   (D) Florence Nightingale is a famous person.

Section II

At this time in history, Florence Nightingale was entering into what was considered by many to be a shady calling with poorly trained, "lower class," workers and exposure to danger, disease, and grossly unpleasant circumstances. Florence perceived a need and set out to change nursing.

12. Which statement summarizes section II?

   (A) There was no such thing as nursing before Florence Nightingale.
   (B) Nursing, before Florence Nightingale, was considered not too inviting a career choice.
   (C) Disease was gross before Florence Nightingale.
   (D) Soldiers were poorly cared for before Florence Nightingale.

Section III

Florence Nightingale first distinguished herself by her work at Scutari in the Crimea during the Crimean War. She demonstrated that general cleanliness, fresh air, use of sanitary food, and maintaining clean water could lessen morbidity, or illness, and could slow mortality, or death rates, among soldiers. For the first time, she demonstrated that treating the British foot soldier as more than a low-level wastrel would lead to successes on many levels.

13. Which of the following is an accurate synopsis of section III?

   (A) At Scutari, Florence Nightingale demonstrated the benefits of a change in attitude and hygiene.
   (B) At Scutari, Florence Nightingale fought alongside the men.
   (C) Although death rates initially rose when Florence Nightingale began work at Scutari, she soon reversed the trend.
   (D) Florence Nightingale was never really at Scutari, although she was present in the Crimea.

14. The respective meanings of *morbidity* and *mortality* are:

   (A) disease and death.
   (B) hunger and starvation.
   (C) death and disease.
   (D) none of the above.

Section IV

After much publicity, Florence Nightingale returned to England and, on the crest of heady popularity, set out to open her school of nursing. She and Elizabeth Blackwell, the first female American physician, met and discussed whether Florence Nightingale's nursing school system should be a stepping stone, for the best trainees, into the world of medical practice. It has been said that Elizabeth Blackwell advocated medical training, leading to a physician's license, for the best of the nursing graduates. Florence Nightingale seems to have felt otherwise. She remained steadfast in her belief that a nurse was a nurse and a physician a physician. Florence Nightingale's views in this area continue to dominate nursing thinking to this day.

15. What is a major theme of section IV?

   (A) Florence Nightingale established training schools and knew and held discussions with Elizabeth Blackwell on those occasions when Florence Nightingale visited America.
   (B) Florence Nightingale remained steadfast in her belief that nursing and medicine should remain separate fields.
   (C) It can be inferred that Florence Nightingale hated Elizabeth Blackwell.
   (D) Florence Nightingale was very angry at the medical establishment for blocking her earlier efforts with soldiers overseas and would never again give credence to their views.

Reading Comprehension Sample Test Answer Key

1. **(D)** Diamonds have a hardness of 10 and will not be affected if an attempt was made to scratch it with a knife. Choices A, B, and C were not mentioned in the discussion of hardness.

2. **(B)** Minerals are known for their chemical composition and physical properties. Minerals are individual in structure. The other choices are incorrect.

3. **(C)** Sedimentary rocks are formed from pieces of other rocks and minerals. A metamorphic rock combined with a sedimentary rock, broken apart through wind and flowing water becomes sediment. The sediment can then be compacted or cemented into a sedimentary rock.

4. **(A)** The theme of the paragraph relates to feeling. Choice A discussed time correlating with living. Individual positive experiences and time get lost in such experiences, and time has a different meaning for each person.

5. **(D)** All paragraphs focus on man and time. Choices A, B, and C are mentioned in other paragraphs, but do not fall into the overall categorical theme.

6. **(C)** Humans live relating time to physical, feeling, and living aspects; that is, as discussed in the paragraph: physics, metaphysics, and ethics, respectively. Although choices A, B, and D may have some relevance for some people, they are not applicable here.

7. **(A)** The initial discussion of Greek history illustrates how man and time has been an issue for centuries. The other choices are unrelated.

8. **(C)** Only choice C explains the example as used in the paragraph. Choices A, B, and D do not relate to the example.

9. **(D)** Rereading the paragraph shows that Fen/Phen was effective, but it damaged the heart, in some cases.

10. **(B)** One would perhaps need to reread the paragraph briefly to find which depressed and which elevated the alertness level.

Timed Reading and Response

Count the number of lines you read at the end of one minute, the point where you would have made your mark. One who reads very quickly would have made it to line 45. One who reads at a more moderate pace would have made it to line 33 or so. If you were slower at reading, you need to practice. And when you are accepted into nursing school, make an effort to attend all lectures because these will sum up content so that you will not need to rely entirely on reading pace for success.

You will recall that you had an initial one-minute session followed by an additional seven minutes. The correct responses for your eight-minute session follow. You should have completed the reading and the questions within the eight-minute total session.

11. **(B)**

12. **(B)**

13. **(A)** Choices B, C, and D were never mentioned or implied in the reading comprehension paragraph.

14. **(A)** Morbidity is disease, and mortality is death.

15. **(B)** One must surmise the strength of Florence Nightingale's belief. Choice A is incorrect since we are not told that Florence Nightingale ever visited America. Choices C and D take the paragraph's message beyond what was stated.

Numerical Ability

The ability to use numbers competently is essential in virtually every aspect of our everyday lives. Numerical ability is nothing more than using mathematics effectively in its many different forms.

We are surrounded by numbers. Consider the following examples that use numbers and require some mathematical ability:

1. You set your alarm clock to get up at a certain time each morning. The time you choose to get up depends on the number of tasks you must accomplish before leaving to get to school or work on time.

2. You purchase a number of items at a store. The clerk tells you the cost of your purchase, and you must know how much money to give to the clerk, as well as how to determine the amount of change you should receive.

3. You want to purchase your first car. You will probably have to see if car payments will fit into your budget. Moreover, a car costs more than the price posted on the window sticker. You must pay for taxes, title, and license as well as the interest on the car loan. You must also see if car insurance will fit into your budget.

4. You decide to paint several rooms in your apartment, so you must determine how many square feet there are to be painted before you can buy the correct amount of paint.

5. You have volunteered to bake 100 dozen chocolate chip cookies for the charity bazaar. Your chocolate chip cookie recipe yields three dozen cookies approximately three inches in diameter. You will need to determine the total amount of ingredients to purchase in order to bake this large amount of cookies.

In nursing, just as in everyday life, good numerical skills are as important as having good communication skills. Nurses use many levels of mathematics from simple arithmetic to more advanced algebra in all aspects of patient care. Consider that nurses are responsible for their own actions, and a nurse with poor numerical ability may harm or kill a patient. For example, a patient may receive medication based on body weight and the nurse is responsible for not only knowing what the patient weighs but also figuring the amount of medication the patient is to receive based on the physician's order. The patient could get too much or too little medication if the nurse's numerical skills were not up to par.

To complicate matters even more, a number of measuring systems are currently in use. In the United States, the English system is commonly used. Much of the rest of the world uses the metric system. The health care system in the United States also uses the metric system.

Converting from the English system of measurement to the metric or from the metric system to the English when you do not know the equivalents can easily be done using the ratio and proportion formula presented later in this chapter. Ratio and proportion can also be used when going from one unit of measure to another within each system. Common metric measurements are presented in Table 5.1.

Table 5.1
Common Metric Measurements

Gram (Mass)[a]	Equivalents in Other Units
1000 mcg	1 mg
1000 mg	1 g
1000 g	1 kg[d]
1000 kg	1 metric ton

Liter (Volume)[b]	Equivalents in Other Units
1000 ml	1 L
1000 L	1 kl

Meter (Length)[c]	Equivalents in Other Units
1000 mm	100 cm
100 cm	10 dm
10 dm	1 m
1 m	10 dam
10 dam	100 hm
100 hm	1000 km

[a]mcg = microgram, mg = milligram, g = gram, kg = kilogram.
[b]ml = milliliter, L = liter, kl = kiloliter.
[c]mm = millimeter, cm = centimeter, dm = decimeter, m = meter, dam = dekameter, hm = hectometer, km = kilometer.
[d]1 kg = 2.2 lbs.

Just as it is difficult to conceive of life without using numbers in one form or another, it is difficult to think of many situations where measurements of one type or another are not used. Measurements are presented in numerical format, and you should be familiar with a number of measurements, many of which are shown in Table 5.2.

Table 5.2
Units of Measurement

Unit	U.S. Equivalent	Metric Equivalent
Length		
foot	12 inches	0.305 meters
yard	3 feet (36 inches)	0.914 meters
rod	5.5 yards	5.029 meters
statute mile	1,760 yards (5,280 feet)	1.609 kilometers
nautical mile	1,151 statute miles	1.852 kilometers
Area		
square foot	144 square inches	929.030 square centimeters
square yard	9 square feet	0.836 square meters
acre	4,840 square yards	4,072 square meters
section	1 square mile (640 acres)	2,590 square kilometers
Capacity		
ounce	8 drams	29.573 milliliters
cup	8 ounces	0.237 liter
pint	16 ounces	0.473 liter
quart	2 pints	0.946 liter
gallon	4 quarts	3.785 liters
peck	8 quarts	8.810 liters
bushel	4 pecks	35.239 liters
Weight		
ounce	16 drams	28.350 grams
pound	16 ounces	0.45 kg (1 kg = 2.21 lbs.)
ton	2,000 pounds	0.907 metric tons

Unit	U.S. and Metric Equivalents
Time	
minute	60 seconds
hour	60 minutes
day	24 hours
year	365 days or 12 months
decade	10 years
century	100 years
millennium	1000 years

Nurses use measurements in numerous aspects of patient care. In many instances nurses use the metric system of measurement. For example, a record may be kept of the amount of fluids a patient takes in orally and the amount of urine a patient puts out. Nurses calculating a patient's intake and output would need to be able to convert from the liquid measurement system to the metric system. Table 5.3 lists the most common nursing measurements.

Table 5.3
Common Nursing Measurements[a]

Household Equivalent	English Equivalent	Metric Equivalent
1 gtt (drop)	1 m (minum)	0.06 ml (milliliter)
	15 or 16 m	1 ml
60 gtt = 1 tsp = 5 ml	1 fluid dram	5 ml
3 tsp = 1 tbsp	4 fluid drams	15 or 16 ml
2 tbsp	1 fluid ounce	30 ml
1 glass = 1 measuring cup	8 fluid ounces = 1/2 pint	240 ml
	1/300 gr	0.2 mg
	1/200 gr	0.3 mg
	1/150 gr	0.4 mg
	1/100 gr	0.6 mg
	1/60 gr	1 mg = 1000 mcg
	1/10 gr	6 mg
	1/8 gr	8 mg
	1/6 gr	10 mg
	1/4 gr	15 mg
	1 gr	60 mg

[a]gtt = drop, m = minum, ml = milliliter, tsp = teaspoon, tbsp = tablespoon, gr = grain, mg = milligram, mcg = microgram.

It is beyond the scope of this book to present all aspects of mathematics, so we assume that you have basic mathematical reasoning abilities and can competently add, subtract, multiply, and divide numbers *without* a calculator.

A number of different mathematical symbols may be used with any type of mathematical problem. You should be familiar with these symbols, which are given in Table 5.4.

Table 5.4
Mathematical Symbols

Symbol	Meaning	Example
+	Add	$10 + 15 = 25$
−	Subtract	$60 - 40 = 20$
$\times$ or $\cdot$ or ( )	Multiply	$6 \times 5 = 30$ or $(6)(5) = 30$
		$7 \cdot 5 = 35$
		$(12)(4) = 48$
$\div$ or $\frac{a}{b}$	Divide	$15 \div 3 = 5$ or $\frac{15}{3} = 5$
		$\frac{50}{5} = 10$
=	Is equal to	$12 = 12$
$\neq$	Is not equal to	$8 \neq 15$
$\geq$	Is equal to or greater than	$a \geq b$
$\leq$	Is equal to or less than	$c \leq d$
>	Is greater than	$7 > 2$
<	Is less than	$9 < 13$
$\perp$	Is perpendicular to	$b \perp d$
$\parallel$	Is parallel to	$a \parallel c$
$\sqrt{\ }$	Square root	$\sqrt{64} = 8$
$\sqrt[3]{\ }$	Cube root	$\sqrt[3]{216} = 6$
( )	Parentheses	$8(6 + 4) = 80$
[ ]	Brackets	$7 + [8(6 + 4) - 2] = 85$
{ }	Braces	$119 + 7 - \{2 + [8(6 + 4) - 8] + 3\} = 49$
$\angle$	Angle	$\angle ABC + 80° = 165°$

Basic Arithmetic Review

Whole Numbers

Whole numbers are composed of digits. Each digit has a place value that helps us "translate" the amount of the number. The American number system is based on ten, and the place or position of each digit indicates what the digit is worth. Figure 5.1 demonstrates our number system using whole and partial numbers. Commas are used as place holders and are placed every three digits beginning with the first whole number to the left of the decimal. Numbers to the left of the decimal are whole numbers, and those to the right are parts of whole numbers in tenths.

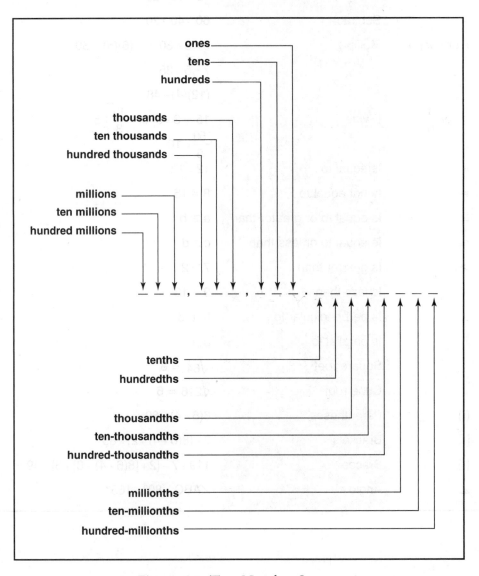

Figure 5.1. Tens Number System

Using the information in Figure 5.1, consider the following examples:

EXAMPLE 1

734,815,690

The 0 is in the ones place and has a value of 1 times 0 or 0. The 9 is in the tens place and has a value of 10 times 9 or 90. The 6 is in the hundreds place and has a value of 100 times 6 or 600. The 5 is in the thousands place and has a value of 1,000 times 5 or 5,000. The 1 is in the ten thousands place and has a value of 10,000 times 1 or 10,000. The 8 is in the hundred thousands place and has a value of 100,000 times 8 or 800,000. The 4 is in the millions place and has a value of 1,000,000 times 4 or 4,000,000, and so on.

EXAMPLE 2

0.6874

The 6 is in the tenths place and has a value of 0.1 times 6 or 0.6. The 8 is in the hundredths place and has a value of 0.01 times 8 or 0.08. The 7 is in the thousandths place and has a value of 0.001 times 7 or .007, and so on.

Number Groupings

Numbers may be grouped by different methods:

- *Natural* or *counting* numbers are 1, 2, 3, 4, 5, 6, . . . , ∞.

- *Whole* numbers are 0, 1, 2, 3, 4, 5, 6, . . . , ∞.

- *Odd* numbers are 1, 3, 5, 7, 9, . . . , ∞. Odd numbers are not divisible by 2.

- *Even* numbers are 0, 2, 4, 6, 8, 10, . . . , ∞. Even numbers are divisible by 2.

- *Rational* numbers are fractions such as $\frac{4}{7}$, $\frac{7}{21}$, and $\frac{10}{6}$.

- *Irrational* numbers are numbers such as $\sqrt{18}$ and π.

- *Prime* numbers can only be evenly divided by 1 and by themselves. Examples of prime numbers include 3, 7, 13, 17, 23, and 31.

- *Composite* numbers are divisible by more than just 1 and themselves. Examples of composite numbers are 2, 6, 10, 15, 21, and 27.

Order of Operations

Mathematical equations are not always clear cut in terms of how to determine the answer to a problem correctly. Determining the answer to equations that are added, subtracted, multiplied, or divided is clear cut. You perform the one operation the problem calls for.

TIP

Mathematical operations must be performed in the prescribed order to obtain a correct answer.

Consider the following equation in which an answer is determined working from the left to the right and ignoring the order of operations:

$$8 + 15 \times 3^2 - 6(4 + 4) =$$

$$23 \times 3^2 - 6(4 + 4) =$$

$$23 \times 9 - 6(4 + 4) =$$

$$207 - 6 \times 8 =$$

$$201 \times 8 = 1,608$$

For problems that contain more than one operation there is an order for performing the different operations encountered. The order of operations is as follows:

Step 1. Perform operations within *parentheses*.

Step 2. Perform operations with powers and *roots*.

Step 3. Beginning on the left of the equation, perform operations requiring *multiplication*.

Step 4. Beginning on the left of the equation, perform operations requiring *division*.

Step 5. Beginning on the left of the equation, perform operations requiring *addition*.

Step 6. Beginning on the left of the equation, perform operations requiring *subtraction*.

When using the order of operations, if one of the steps or operations is not indicated, skip to the next. Let's consider the same equation, only this time use the order of operations to determine the answer:

Equation: $8 + 15 \times 3^2 - 6(4 + 4) =$

Step 1: $8 + 15 \times 3^2 - 6(8) =$

Step 2: $8 + 15 \times 9 - 6(8) =$

Step 3: $8 + 135 - 48 =$

Step 4: No division required.

Step 5: $143 - 48 =$

Step 6: 95

You can see there is a difference in answer when the correct order of operations is followed.

Rounding Numbers

When performing mathematical operations, numbers or answers do not always come out as whole numbers and it may be necessary to round to a whole number. For example, at the end of a course a student has an average of 79.6 percent, but the school's grading system indicates that only whole numbers in the form of percentages may be issued as course grades. What grade does the teacher issue? The average is higher than the next lowest whole number 79, but lower than the next highest whole number of 80. Rounding 79.6 percent allows the teacher to issue a grade of 80 percent.

Rules regarding rounding work with numbers to the left as well as to the right of the decimal place. When rounding numbers, use the following steps:

Step 1. Determine the place value of the number to be rounded. Circle or underline this number.

Step 2. Look at the number immediately to the right of your circled or underlined number.

   A. If that number is 5 or greater, round the circled or underlined number up one place value.

   B. If that number is 4 or smaller, leave the circled or underlined number as it is.

EXAMPLES

Round to the nearest one.

45.87 = 45.81 = 46

13.49 = 13.49 = 13

Round to the nearest ten.

78.149 = 78.149 = 80

2,963.3888 = 2,963.3888 = 2,960

Round to the nearest hundredth.

587.887 = 587.887 = 587.89

13,629.74 = 13,629.740 = 13,629.74

Round to the nearest thousandth.

5.89765 = 5.89765 = 5.898

23.37449 = 23.37449 = 23.374

Positive and Negative Numbers

The value of a number may be positive or negative. Any number preceded by a plus or minus sign may also be referred to as a signed number. On a number line, all numbers to the right of zero are positive, and all numbers to the left of zero are negative.

Positive numbers may be written in two different formats. The first with a plus sign preceding the number, such as +4 or +3.76, and the second simply as the number, such as 14 or 10.13. Negative numbers are always written with a minus sign preceding the number, such as − 38 or − 43.4. When working with both positive and negative numbers in the same equation, positive numbers always display the plus (+) sign before the number. See Figure 5.2.

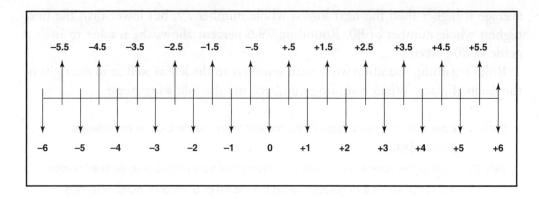

Figure 5.2. Positive/Negative Number Line

There are rules for working with positive and negative numbers that deal with mathematical operations of addition, subtraction, multiplication, and division.

ADDITION

1. When adding numbers with the same sign, perform the operation. Do not change the sign of the sum.

$$+3 + 7 = +10 \qquad\qquad -17 + (-5) = -22$$

2. When adding numbers with different signs, subtract the smaller number from the larger number. Place the sign of the larger number before the sum.

$$-34 + 18 = -16 \qquad\qquad 88 + (-100) = -12$$

SUBTRACTION

1. When subtracting positive numbers, negative numbers, or numbers with different signs, change the sign of the subtrahend (the number being subtracted), then add the numbers together. Place the sign of the minuend (top or first number) before the difference.

$$+84 - (+15) = +84 + (-15) = +69$$

$$-43 - (-11) = -43 + (+11) = -32$$

$$+10 - (-6) = +10 + (+6) = +16$$

$$-23 - (+15) = -23 + (-15) = -38$$

MULTIPLICATION

1. Multiply positive numbers, negative numbers, or numbers with different signs as if they were all positive numbers. The number of negative signs in the equation will determine the sign of the product. Place a *positive* sign before the product if there is an even number of similar signs in the equation. Place a *negative* sign before the product if there is an odd number of odd signs in the equation.

$$(-7)(+4)(+3)(-2) = +168$$

$$(+5)(-2)(-3)(+2)(-2) = -120$$

DIVISION

1. Divide positive numbers, negative numbers, or numbers with different signs as if they were all positive numbers. The number of negative signs in the equation will determine the sign of the quotient. Place a *positive* sign before the quotient if there is an even number of odd signs in the equation. Place a *negative* sign before the quotient if there is an odd number of odd signs in the equation.

$$-14 \div (-2) = +7$$

$$[(-4)(-3)(+2)] \div (+2)(-3) = -4$$

Fractions

Fractions are parts of a whole and are composed of two segments. The numerator, the number before or above the dividing line, tells how many parts are available, and the denominator, the number after or below the dividing line, tells how many pieces are in the whole.

TYPES OF FRACTIONS

Proper fractions are fractions in which the numerator is smaller than the denominator. A proper fraction is less than one whole.

EXAMPLE 1

$$\frac{6}{42} \qquad \frac{15}{100}$$

Improper fractions are fractions in which the numerator is equal to or larger than the denominator. An improper fraction is equal to one whole or more than one whole.

EXAMPLE 2

$$\frac{8}{5} \qquad \frac{42}{7}$$

Mixed numbers are composed of a natural number and a fraction. Mixed numbers are greater than one whole.

EXAMPLE 3

$$2\frac{4}{5} \qquad 16\frac{32}{72}$$

REDUCING FRACTIONS

Reducing a fraction to its lowest terms means dividing the numerator and denominator by a number that divides evenly into both.

EXAMPLE 4

$$\frac{5}{10} = \frac{5 \div 5}{10 \div 5} = \frac{1}{2} \qquad \frac{32}{48} = \frac{32 \div 16}{48 \div 16} = \frac{2}{3}$$

RAISING FRACTIONS

Raising a fraction to higher terms is the opposite of reducing a fraction to its lowest terms. Both the numerator and denominator are multiplied by the same number.

EXAMPLE 5

$$\frac{3}{4} = \frac{3 \cdot 5}{4 \cdot 5} = \frac{15}{20} \qquad \frac{15}{34} = \frac{15 \cdot 2}{34 \cdot 2} = \frac{30}{68}$$

FACTORS

Whole numbers are composed of factors. Factors are numbers that, when multiplied together, equal the whole number. Some numbers have numerous factors whereas others have only one or two.

EXAMPLE 6

The factors of 36 are 1, 2, 3, 4, 6, 9, 12, 18, and 36.

$$36 = 1 \times 36$$
$$= 2 \times 18$$
$$= 3 \times 12$$
$$= 4 \times 9$$
$$= 6 \times 6$$

The factors of 81 are 1, 3, 9, 27, and 81.

$$81 = 1 \times 81$$
$$= 3 \times 27$$
$$= 9 \times 9$$

COMMON FACTORS

Common factors are those factors that are common to two or more whole numbers.

EXAMPLE 7

The common factors of 6, 10, and 12 are 1 and 2. One and 2 are the only factors common to all three numbers.

$$6 = \underline{1} \times 6$$
$$= \underline{2} \times 3$$
$$10 = \underline{1} \times 10$$
$$= \underline{2} \times 5$$
$$12 = \underline{1} \times 12$$
$$= \underline{2} \times 6$$
$$= 3 \times 4$$

The greatest common factor of 6, 10, and 12 is 2; the lowest common factor is 1.

CONVERTING IMPROPER FRACTIONS INTO WHOLE OR MIXED NUMBERS

Improper fractions are converted into whole or mixed numbers by dividing the denominator into the numerator.

EXAMPLE 8

$$\frac{18}{15} = 1\frac{3}{15} = 1\frac{1}{5} \qquad\qquad \frac{100}{50} = 2$$

CONVERTING MIXED NUMBERS INTO IMPROPER FRACTIONS

Mixed numbers are converted into improper fractions by multiplying the denominator of the fraction times the whole number and adding the numerator. This total becomes the new numerator and is placed over the original denominator.

EXAMPLE 9

$$6\frac{2}{5} = \frac{32}{5} \qquad\qquad 17\frac{4}{7} = \frac{123}{7}$$

ADDING FRACTIONS

To add fractions, you must be sure that the denominators of all fractions in the equation are the same. To do this, the lowest common denominator (LCD) of each fraction must be determined. The LCD is the smallest number that divides evenly into all denominators. After you determine the LCD, add the numerators but do not add the denominators. They remain the same.

EXAMPLE 10

$$\frac{5}{8} + \frac{3}{4} = \frac{5}{8} + \frac{6}{8} = \frac{11}{8} \text{ or } 1\frac{3}{8}$$

$$\frac{1}{3} + \frac{3}{7} + \frac{4}{63} = \frac{21}{63} + \frac{27}{63} + \frac{4}{63} = \frac{52}{63}$$

$$3\frac{4}{5} + \frac{1}{10} = 3\frac{8}{10} + \frac{1}{10} = 3\frac{9}{10}$$

SUBTRACTING FRACTIONS

Subtracting fractions is similar to adding fractions. You must determine the LCD before you can subtract.

EXAMPLE 11

$$\frac{7}{8} - \frac{1}{3} = \frac{21}{24} - \frac{8}{24} = \frac{13}{24}$$

$$\frac{3}{5} - \frac{1}{10} = \frac{6}{10} - \frac{1}{10} = \frac{5}{10} \; or \; \frac{1}{2}$$

$$7\frac{2}{3} - 2\frac{1}{5} = 7\frac{10}{15} - 2\frac{3}{15} = 5\frac{7}{15}$$

MULTIPLYING FRACTIONS OR MIXED NUMBERS

To multiply fractions or mixed numbers, you need to multiply the numerators together and then multiply the denominators together.

EXAMPLE 12

$$\frac{4}{5} \cdot \frac{3}{7} = \frac{12}{35}$$

$$\frac{8}{15} \cdot \frac{1}{4} = \frac{8}{60} \; or \; \frac{2}{15}$$

$$8\frac{2}{3} \times \frac{2}{7} = \frac{26}{3} \times \frac{2}{7} = \frac{52}{21} \; or \; 2\frac{10}{21}$$

DIVIDING FRACTIONS

Dividing fractions is similar to multiplying fractions, but it requires an additional step. To divide fractions, you need to invert the fraction you are dividing by and then multiply the two fractions together.

EXAMPLE 13

$$\frac{4}{15} \div \frac{3}{10} = \frac{4}{15} \times \frac{10}{3} = \frac{40}{45} \; or \; \frac{8}{9}$$

$$17 \div \frac{3}{4} = \frac{17}{1} \times \frac{4}{3} = \frac{68}{3} = 22\frac{2}{3}$$

DECIMALS

Decimals and fractions have a very special relationship because decimals are a type of fraction. If you discount the previous section on fractions, the majority of our discussion on numerical ability has dealt with numbers to the left of the decimal in our tens numbering system. We have been talking about whole numbers.

Decimals refer to numbers to the right of the decimal in our tens numbering system. Look back at Figure 5.1 if you need to review; then consider Table 5.5. Notice that the denominators of the fractions are in tens, which is 1×10; then 100, which is 10×10; then 1,000, which is 100×10; and so on.

Table 5.5
Decimals and Fractions

Places to the Right of the Decimal	Name	Example	Fraction
One	Tenths	0.3	$\frac{3}{10}$
Two	Hundredths	0.87	$\frac{87}{100}$
Three	Thousandths	0.231	$\frac{231}{1,000}$
Four	Ten-thousandths	0.4543	$\frac{4543}{10,000}$
Five	Hundred-thousandths	0.18766	$\frac{18,766}{100,000}$
Six	Millionths	0.241296	$\frac{241,296}{1,000,000}$

CHANGING FRACTIONS TO DECIMALS

Fractions may be changed into decimals by dividing the denominator into the numerator.

EXAMPLE 1

$$\frac{3}{4} = 0.75$$
$$\frac{7}{8} = 0.875$$

CHANGING DECIMALS TO FRACTIONS

When changing a decimal to a fraction, note the number of places to the right of the decimal to determine the name of the decimal. This determines the denominator of your fraction. Then change the number to a whole number, and use it as the numerator in your fraction.

EXAMPLE 2

$$0.84 = \frac{85}{100}$$

$$0.675 = \frac{675}{1,000}$$

ADDING OR SUBTRACTING DECIMALS

Adding or subtracting decimals is no different from adding or subtracting other numbers except that the decimal points must be aligned. As with using the orders of operation, you must follow the rules. You will get an incorrect answer if the decimals are not aligned.

EXAMPLE 3

```
  4,755.000
     18.870          87.704
     32.987         -16.440
     16.400          71.264
 +  187.040
  5,010.297
```

MULTIPLYING DECIMALS

Multiplying decimals is no different than multiplying other numbers, except that you must take the decimal places into account. Multiply the numbers in the regular fashion. Your answer is a whole number. Count the number of decimal places in the multiplicand and multiplier (the top and bottom numbers). Then count over from the right of the product the number of places that totals the decimal places in the multiplicand and multiplier.

EXAMPLE 4

$$806.12$$
$$\times 17.334$$
$$\overline{13,973.28408}$$

$$10$$
$$\times 10.14$$
$$\overline{101.40}$$

DIVIDING DECIMALS

Dividing decimals is no different than dividing any other numbers, except that, once again, you must take the decimals into account before you start to divide. The divisor (the number being divided into another number) must be a whole number. The number of decimal places in the divisor must be moved to the right until you have a whole number. The number of spaces the decimal is moved to the right is the same number of spaces the decimal will be moved to the right in the dividend (the number being divided into). Moving the decimals in the divisor and the dividend will always make them larger numbers.

EXAMPLE 5

$$3.2\overline{)36.0} = 32\overline{)\overset{11.25}{360.00}}$$

$$103.06\overline{)488.693} = 10,306\overline{)\overset{4.7418}{48,869.3000}}$$

PERCENTAGE

Percents are another form of fractions. Percents are unique in that the denominator is always 100 in the fraction form. The percent sign (%) is used instead of 100 and stands for per hundred. In most cases, 100% is the totality of something. It is possible to have more than 100% of something. If a business increased its profits from $1 million in one year to $5 million the next year, the increase in profits is 500%.

CHANGING A DECIMAL TO A PERCENT AND BACK AGAIN

Move the decimal place two spaces to the right to change a decimal to a percent. The decimal moves in the opposite direction to change a percent to a decimal.

EXAMPLE 1

$$0.47 = 47\% = 0.47$$

$$0.6012 = 60.12\% = 0.6012$$

$$87 \text{ or } 87.00 = 8700\% = 87$$

CHANGING A FRACTION TO A PERCENT AND BACK AGAIN

Changing a fraction to a percent involves two steps. First, you must change the fraction into a decimal, and then change the decimal into a percent. Changing a percent to a fraction runs through these steps backwards. Change the percent to a decimal, change the decimal to a fraction, and then reduce as necessary.

EXAMPLE 2

$$\frac{3}{4} = 0.75 = 75\% = 0.75 = \frac{3}{4}$$

$$\frac{13}{51} = 0.2549 = 25.49\% = 0.2549 = \frac{13}{51}$$

Learning the equivalents can save time and energy. Table 5.6 contains equivalents you should be familiar with.

TIP

Memorize these equivalents. They will save time when calculating problems.

Table 5.6
Fraction-Decimal-Percentage Equivalents

Fraction	Decimal	Percentage
$\frac{1}{4}$	0.25	25%
$\frac{1}{2}$	0.50	50%
$\frac{3}{4}$	0.75	75%
$\frac{1}{3}$	$0.33\frac{1}{3}$ or $0.33\overline{3}$	$33.\overline{3}$%
$\frac{2}{3}$	$0.66\frac{2}{3}$ or $0.66\overline{6}$	$66.\overline{6}$%
$\frac{1}{5}$	0.20	20%
$\frac{3}{5}$	0.60	60%
$\frac{4}{5}$	0.80	80%
$\frac{1}{6}$	$0.16\frac{2}{3}$ or $0.16\overline{6}$	$16.\overline{6}$%
$\frac{5}{6}$	$0.83\frac{1}{3}$ or $0.83\overline{3}$	$83.\overline{3}$%
$\frac{1}{8}$	0.125	12.5%
$\frac{3}{8}$	0.375	37.5%
$\frac{5}{8}$	0.625	62.5%
$\frac{7}{8}$	0.875	87.5%

Exponents and Powers

An exponent indicates that a number must be multiplied by itself a number of times. It can be either a positive or negative number. The number to be multiplied by itself is called the base, and the exponent is a superscript number to the right of the base. In example one, the bases are 5, 7, 4, and 8, and 2, 6, –4, and –3 are exponents.

EXAMPLE 1

$$5^2 = 5 \times 5 = 25$$
$$7^6 = 7 \times 7 \times 7 \times 7 \times 7 \times 7 = 117,649$$
$$4^{-4} = \frac{1}{4^4} = \frac{1}{4 \times 4 \times 4 \times 4} = \frac{1}{256}$$
$$8^{-3} = \frac{1}{8^3} = \frac{1}{8 \times 8 \times 8} = \frac{1}{512}$$

The following rules apply to exponents:

1. When adding or subtracting exponents with the same or different bases, each base with an exponent must be simplified before the addition or subtraction can take place.

EXAMPLE 2

$$6^3 + 2^4 = 216 + 16 = 232$$
$$8^2 + 4^6 = 64 + 4096 = 4160$$
$$5^3 - 3^2 = 125 - 9 = 116$$
$$7^5 - 7^3 = 16,807 - 343 = 16,464$$

2. When multiplying or dividing exponents with different bases, each base must be simplified before the multiplication or division can take place.

EXAMPLE 3

$$8^4 \times 2^7 = 4096 \times 128 = 524,288$$
$$4^3 \div 2^3 = 64 \div 8 = 8$$
$$6^3 \div 5^3 = 216 \div 125 = 1.728$$

3. Multiply the exponents when raising a power to another power.

EXAMPLE 4

$$(9^5)^2 = 9^{5 \times 2} = 9^{10}$$
$$(2^4)^3 = 2^{4 \times 3} = 2^{12}$$

4. Add the exponents when multiplying powers with the same nonzero bases.

EXAMPLE 5

$$3^4 \times 3^2 = 3^{4+2} = 3^6$$

$$7^3 \times 7^2 \times 7^7 = 7^{3+2+7} = 7^{12}$$

---

5. Subtract the exponents when dividing powers with the same nonzero bases.

EXAMPLE 6

$$4^9 \div 4^6 = \frac{4^9}{4^6} = 4^{9-6} = 4^3$$

$$8^5 \div 8^2 = \frac{8^5}{8^2} = 8^{5-2} = 8^3$$

You should be familiar with the square and cube numbers listed in Table 5.7.

Table 5.7
Square and Cube Numbers

Whole Number	Number Squared	Number Cubed
0	0	0
1	1	1
2	4	8
3	9	27
4	16	64
5	25	125
6	36	216
7	49	343
8	64	512
9	81	729
10	100	1,000
11	121	1,331
12	144	1,728

Square Roots and Cube Roots

There is a relationship between powers and roots. The square of a number is the product of a number multiplied by itself, or twice. The cube of a number is the product of a number multiplied by itself three times.

In $\sqrt{81}$, the $\sqrt{}$ is the radical and 81 is the radicand. When finding the square root of a radicand, you are interested in finding a number that when multiplied by itself equals the radicand. When finding the cube root of a radicand, you are interested in finding a number that when multiplied by itself three times, or cubed, equals the radicand.

EXAMPLE 1

$$\sqrt{81} = 9 = \sqrt{9 \times 9}$$

$$\sqrt{34} = 5.8309 = \sqrt{5.8309 \times 5.8309}$$

$$\sqrt[3]{27} = 3 = \sqrt{3 \times 3 \times 3}$$

$$\sqrt[3]{216} = 6 = \sqrt{6 \times 6 \times 6}$$

Simple Statistics

Simple statistics deals with means, medians, and modes. The mean, also called the average, is determined by adding a series of items or numbers and dividing by the number of items.

EXAMPLE 1

Determine the mean of the numbers 5, 10, 22, and 7.

$$5 + 10 + 22 + 7 = 44 \div 4 = 11.$$

The average of the set of numbers is 11.

The median is the middle number in a set of numbers arranged in ascending or descending order. With an odd set of numbers the median is always the middle number. If there is an even set of numbers, the median is the average of the two middle numbers.

EXAMPLE 2

Determine the median of the following set of numbers: 5, 10, 6, 15, 12, 8, 1, and 22.

1, 5, 6, 8, 10, 12, 15, 22

$$8 + 10 = 18 \div 2 = 9$$

The median of the set of numbers is 9.

The mode is the number that occurs most often in a series of numbers.

EXAMPLE 3

Determine the mode of the following set of numbers: 3, 7, 9, 16, 16, 18, 22, 54.

The mode of the set of numbers is 16.

Answer Sheet
SAMPLE TEST

Basic Arithmetic

1 Ⓐ Ⓑ Ⓒ Ⓓ   10 Ⓐ Ⓑ Ⓒ Ⓓ   19 Ⓐ Ⓑ Ⓒ Ⓓ
2 Ⓐ Ⓑ Ⓒ Ⓓ   11 Ⓐ Ⓑ Ⓒ Ⓓ   20 Ⓐ Ⓑ Ⓒ Ⓓ
3 Ⓐ Ⓑ Ⓒ Ⓓ   12 Ⓐ Ⓑ Ⓒ Ⓓ   21 Ⓐ Ⓑ Ⓒ Ⓓ
4 Ⓐ Ⓑ Ⓒ Ⓓ   13 Ⓐ Ⓑ Ⓒ Ⓓ   22 Ⓐ Ⓑ Ⓒ Ⓓ
5 Ⓐ Ⓑ Ⓒ Ⓓ   14 Ⓐ Ⓑ Ⓒ Ⓓ   23 Ⓐ Ⓑ Ⓒ Ⓓ
6 Ⓐ Ⓑ Ⓒ Ⓓ   15 Ⓐ Ⓑ Ⓒ Ⓓ   24 Ⓐ Ⓑ Ⓒ Ⓓ
7 Ⓐ Ⓑ Ⓒ Ⓓ   16 Ⓐ Ⓑ Ⓒ Ⓓ   25 Ⓐ Ⓑ Ⓒ Ⓓ
8 Ⓐ Ⓑ Ⓒ Ⓓ   17 Ⓐ Ⓑ Ⓒ Ⓓ
9 Ⓐ Ⓑ Ⓒ Ⓓ   18 Ⓐ Ⓑ Ⓒ Ⓓ

Basic Arithmetic Sample Test

Basic Arithmetic Sample Test

Directions: For each question, select the letter (A, B, C, or D) that corresponds to your answer. Record your answers on the answer sheet on page 131.

1. $6 + 14 - 3(4 + 2) + 2(5^2 - 15) =$

   (A) 35
   (B) 22
   (C) 18
   (D) 58

2. Identify the unique characteristic of the following odd numbers: 3, 7, 13, 21, 59, and 87.

   (A) They are divisible by 3 or 7.
   (B) They are rational numbers.
   (C) They are not divisible by 2.
   (D) They are not prime numbers.

3. Identify the average of the following numbers: 15, 18, 4, 22, 38, 56.

   (A) 6
   (B) 25.5
   (C) 159
   (D) 918

4. Identify the rational number: CHALLENGE

   $\sqrt{64}$ $\dfrac{7}{32}$ 8 π

   (A) π

   (B) $\sqrt{64}$

   (C) 8

   (D) $\dfrac{7}{32}$

5. Identify the number in the tenths place: 347.1896

   (A) 7
   (B) 9
   (C) 4
   (D) 1

6. $13 - 2^3 + 4(3 - 1) =$

   (A) 13
   (B) 17
   (C) 16
   (D) 2

7. $-45 + (-7) =$

   (A) 38
   (B) -38
   (C) 52
   (D) -52

8. $-35 \div 5 + 8^2(5 - 3) =$ CHALLENGE

   (A) 135
   (B) 121
   (C) 249
   (D) 505

9. Factors common to 15 and 30 are

   (A) 1, 3, 5, 15.
   (B) 1, 3, 5, 10.
   (C) 2, 3, 5, 15.
   (D) 3, 5, 6, 10.

10. $\dfrac{7}{10} + \dfrac{3}{20} =$

   (A) $\dfrac{13}{20}$

   (B) $\dfrac{17}{20}$

   (C) $\dfrac{10}{30}$ or $\dfrac{1}{3}$

   (D) 1

11. $\frac{15}{100} =$

 (A) 150%
 (B) 15%
 (C) 1.5%
 (D) .15%

12. $(17.412)(3.78) =$

 (A) 63.42170
 (B) 51.0
 (C) 65.81
 (D) 65.81736

13. $0.7424 =$

 (A) 74.24%
 (B) 7424%
 (C) 7.424%
 (D) 80.0%

14. $4^3 + 2^5 =$

 (A) 6^8
 (B) 96
 (C) 36
 (D) 6^{-2}

15. $\sqrt{144} =$

 (A) 11
 (B) 14.4
 (C) 12
 (D) 14

16. $\sqrt[3]{64} - 4(15 - 4) + 7^2 - (-14 + 14) =$

 (A) 13   **CHALLENGE**
 (B) 41
 (C) 5.7
 (D) 9

17. $\frac{5}{7} \div 3\frac{4}{5} =$

 (A) 2.714
 (B) 0.18797
 (C) 38.6114
 (D) 1.896

18. $15^3 =$

 (A) 45
 (B) 5
 (C) 3375
 (D) 18

19. 58% of 17 yards =

 (A) 29 inches
 (B) 110 inches
 (C) 118.32 inches
 (D) 355 inches

20. $857.42 \div 7.056 =$

 (A) 121.52
 (B) 0.121516
 (C) 0.0082
 (D) 122.42

21. $6^{-4} =$

 (A) $\frac{1}{1296}$
 (B) -1296
 (C) -4
 (D) -24

22. $\frac{3}{4}(7 + 13) \div [4(3 \times 2) + 15] =$

 (A) 15.625   **CHALLENGE**
 (B) 585
 (C) 0.3846
 (D) 11.875

23. 2 square miles =

 (A) 4,840 acres
 (B) 1,280 acres
 (C) 2,590 acres
 (D) 929.3 acres

24. 4 pecks =

 (A) 8 quarts
 (B) 3 quarts
 (C) 32 quarts
 (D) 20 quarts

25. Determine the median of the following numbers: 10, 15, 39, 8, 17, 27, and 21.

 (A) 8
 (B) 32
 (C) 7
 (D) 17

Basic Arithmetic Sample Test Answer Key

1. **(B)** $6 + 14 - 3(4 + 2) + 2(5^2 - 15)$
   $= 6 + 14 - 3(6) + 2(10)$
   $= 6 + 14 - 18 + 20$
   $= 40 - 18 = 22$

2. **(C)** They are not divisible by 2. Only even numbers are divisible by 2.

3. **(B)** $(15 + 18 + 4 + 22 + 38 + 56) = 153 \div 6 = 25.5$

4. **(D)** Fractions are rational numbers.

5. **(D)** 347.$\underline{1}$896

6. **(A)** $13 - 2^3 + 4(3 - 1)$
   $= 13 - 2^3 + 4(2)$
   $= 13 - 8 + 4(2)$
   $= 13 - 8 + 8$
   $= 21 - 8 = 13$

7. **(D)** $-45 + (-7) = -45 - 7 = -52$

8. **(B)** $-35 \div 5 + 8^2(5 - 3)$
   $= -35 \div 5 + 8^2(2)$
   $= -35 \div 5 + 64(2)$
   $= -35 \div 5 + 128$
   $= -7 + 128 = 121$

9. **(A)** $15 = \underline{1} \times \underline{15}$ $30 = \underline{1} \times 30$
   $ = \underline{3} \times \underline{5}$ $= 2 \times \underline{15}$
   $ = \underline{3} \times 10$
   $ = \underline{5} \times 6$

10. **(B)** $\dfrac{7}{10} + \dfrac{3}{20} = \dfrac{14}{20} + \dfrac{3}{20} = \dfrac{17}{20}$

11. **(B)** $\dfrac{15}{100} = 0.15 = 15\%$

12. **(D)** After multiplying the two numbers, count over five decimal places to the left to determine correct answer.

13. **(A)** $0.7424 = 74.24\%$

14. **(B)** $4^3 + 2^5 = 64 + 32 = 96$

15. **(C)** $\sqrt{144} = \sqrt{12 \times 12}$

Basic Arithmetic Sample Test

16. **(D)** $\sqrt[3]{64} - 4(15 - 4) + 7^2 - (-14 + 14)$

$= \sqrt[3]{64} - 4(11) + 7^2 - (0)$
$= 4 - 4(11) + 49$
$= 4 - 44 + 49 = 9$

17. **(B)** $\dfrac{5}{7} \div 3\dfrac{4}{5} = \dfrac{5}{7} \times \dfrac{5}{19} = \dfrac{25}{133} = 0.18797$

18. **(C)** $15^3 = 15 \times 15 \times 15 = 3{,}375$

19. **(D)** 1 yard = 36 inches
17×36 inches = 612 inches
58% of 612 inches = 0.58×612
= 354.96 inches = 355 inches

20. **(A)** $7.056\overline{)857.42} =$

$\dfrac{121.5164399}{7056\overline{)857420.0000000}} = 121.52$

21. **(A)** $6^{-4} = \dfrac{1}{6^4} = \dfrac{1}{6 \times 6 \times 6 \times 6} = \dfrac{1}{1{,}296}$

22. **(C)** $\dfrac{3}{4}(7 + 13) \div [4\,(3 \times 2) + 15]$

$= 0.75(20) \div [4(6) + 15]$
$= 15 \div [24 + 15]$
$= 15 \div 39$
$= 0.3846153 = 0.3846$

23. **(B)** 1 square mile = 640 acres
2×640 acres = 1,280 acres

24. **(C)** 1 peck = 8 quarts
4×8 quarts = 32 quarts

25. **(D)** 8, 10, 15, <u>17</u>, 21, 27, 39

Basic Arithmetic Sample Test

Algebra Review

Algebra is similar to arithmetic except that letters are used in the place of some numbers. Much of algebra has to do with solving an equation or an algebraic expression. When solving such an expression, you must find the value of one or more components of the expression. These components, called variables, are generally identified as x or y, but other letters may be used. Variables are equal to a number. The following are algebraic expressions:

$$3a - 5 = 10$$

$$5(x^3 + 4) - x^2 + 3 = 4x$$

$$\frac{3}{4}y + 15 - y = 45$$

$$2(5x + 5) \div 2x^2 - 7 = 0$$

Evaluating Algebraic Expressions

When evaluating algebraic expressions, replace the letters in the expression with their known numerical value; then solve the expression.

EXAMPLE 1

Evaluate $2x + 3y - x^2$, if $x = 5$ and $y = 10$.

$2(5) + 3(10) - 5^2 = 10 + 30 - 25 = 40 - 25 = 15$

In this example the x with $2x$ cannot be combined with the x^2 because they have different exponents. Only variables with like exponents can be combined.

EXAMPLE 2

Evaluate $4 + 8(a + 6) \div b^2$, if $a = 10$ and $b = 2$.

$4 + 8(10 + 6) \div 2^2 = 4 + 8(16) \div 4 = 4 + 128 \div 4 = 132 \div 4 = 33$

Solving Equations with Inverse Operations

Algebra has mathematical sentences just as grammatical sentences do. The difference is that mathematical sentences use numbers and letters, whereas grammatical sentences use words and numbers. Mathematical sentences are called equations, and an equation tells us that the two sides of the equation are equal.

The equal sign (=) is important in algebra because it indicates that each side of the equation must be equal as the equation is solved. Consequently, what you do to one side of the equal sign in the equation you must also do to the other side of the equal sign in the equation. Prior to solving an algebraic equation, the unknown variable must be isolated on one side of the equation. The remaining information or constant should be placed on the other side of the equation.

EXAMPLE 1

$3x-5=10$	$4+5a-4=30$
$3x=15$	$5a=30$
$x=5$	$a=6$

After you have solved an algebraic equation, you can replace the letters with the numbers, and one side of the equation should equal the other. This is how you check your answers in algebra.

EXAMPLE 2

$3x-5=15$	$3x-5=15$
$3x=20$	$3(6.66)-5=15$
$x=6.66$	$20-5=15$
	$15=15$
$x+17=30$	$x+17=30$
$x=30-17$	$13+17=30$
$x=13$	$30=30$

There are a number of rules for solving algebraic equations. As with other orders of operation, the rules must be followed in order to obtain the correct answer.

1. Remove all grouping symbols, such as parentheses and brackets. Perform the addition, subtraction, multiplication, or division inside of the groupings prior to removing the grouping symbols.

EXAMPLE 3

$$5(x-3)-3=30$$
$$5x-15-3=30$$
$$5x-18=30$$
$$5x=48$$
$$x=9.6$$

$$5(x-3)-3=30$$
$$5(9.6-3)-3=30$$
$$5(6.6)-3=30$$
$$33-3=30$$
$$30=30$$

2. Change fractions into whole numbers using the least common denominator of the fractions before solving the equation. Then combine like terms on each side of the equation.

EXAMPLE 4

$$\frac{1}{2}(x+1)+\frac{3}{5}(x+2)=0$$

$$\left(\frac{1}{10}\right)\frac{1}{2}(x+1)+\left(\frac{10}{1}\right)\frac{3}{5}(x+2)=0\left(\frac{10}{1}\right)$$

$$5(x+1)+6(x+2)=0$$

$$5x+5+6x+12=0$$

$$11x+17=0$$

$$11x=-17$$

$$x=-1.545$$

$$\frac{1}{2}(x+1)+\frac{3}{5}(x+2)=0$$

$$5(-1.545+1)+6(-1.545+2)=0$$

$$5(-0.545)+6(0.0455)=0$$

$$-2.73+2.73=0$$

$$0=0$$

3. Starting at the left side of the expression, perform all operations involving multiplication and division. Then moving from the left side of the expression, perform all operations involving addition and subtraction.

EXAMPLE 5

$$4(6x+10)-3[(3x+7)-(2x-3)]=160$$

$$24x+40-3(x+10)=160$$

$$24x+40-3x-30=160$$

$$21x+10=160$$

$$21x=150$$

$$x=7.14$$

$$4(6x+10)-3[(3x+7)-(2x-3)]=160$$

$$4(52.84)-3[(28.42)-(11.28)]=160$$

$$4(52.84)-3(17.14)=160$$

$$211.36-51.42=160$$

$$160=160$$

$$5b+2[(b+17)+(2b-5)]=50$$

$$5b+2(3b+12)=50$$

$$5b+6b+24=50$$

$$11b=26$$

$$b=2.36$$

$$5b+2[(b+17)+(2b-5)]=50$$

$$5(2.36)+2[(19.36)+(-0.28)]=50$$

$$11.8+2(19.08)=50$$

$$11.8+36.18=50$$

$$50=50$$

4. Cross multiply if the equation states that one fraction is equal to another fraction. Then solve the problem. Cross multiplying means multiplying the numerator of the first side of the equation with the denominator of the second side of the equation, and multiplying the denominator of the first side of the equation with the numerator of the second side of the equation.

EXAMPLE 6

$$\frac{5}{8} = \frac{x}{40} \qquad\qquad \frac{5}{8} = \frac{x}{40}$$

$$8x = 200 \qquad\qquad \frac{5}{8} = \frac{25}{40}$$

$$x = 25 \qquad\qquad \frac{5}{8} = \frac{5}{8}$$

$$\frac{1}{2} = \frac{a}{50} \qquad\qquad \frac{1}{2} = \frac{a}{50}$$

$$2a = 50 \qquad\qquad \frac{1}{2} = \frac{25}{50}$$

$$a = 25 \qquad\qquad \frac{1}{2} = \frac{1}{2}$$

Ratio and Proportion

Ratios are numbers that have something in common. They have some type of relationship. Ratios compare two numbers, and may be written in one of two formats:

$$x : y \text{ or } \frac{x}{y}$$

Both are read "x is to y" with the variable following the "to" as the denominator in the fraction.

EXAMPLE 1

$$6 : 8 \qquad \frac{6}{8}$$

$$50 : 1 \qquad \frac{50}{1}$$

Proportions are two ratios that are equal to each other. In proportion problems, there is usually one variable that is not known and must be determined. Proportions are written in a format similar to the ratio format.

EXAMPLE 2

$$a:b=c:d \text{ or } \frac{a}{b}=\frac{c}{d}$$

The problem is read *a* is to *b* as *c* is to *d*.

$$4:8=3:18 \text{ or } \frac{4}{8}=\frac{3}{18}$$

The problem is read four is to eight as three is to eighteen.

When solving proportion problems, the format you use will determine how you go about solving the problem. Either format is acceptable and both will give the correct answer.

EXAMPLE 3

Solve for *x* in this proportion: 5 is to 10 as *x* is to 20.

With the linear format, you multiply the means or numbers nearest the equal sign, and multiply the extremes or the numbers on the outside of the problem.

$$5:10=x:20$$

$$(10)(x)=(5)(20)$$

$$10x=100$$

$$x=10$$

Utilizing the fractions format, you cross multiply and then solve the problem.

$$\frac{5}{10}=\frac{x}{20}$$

$$(10)(x)=(5)(20)$$

$$10x=100$$

$$x=10$$

Both algebra and geometry use various formulas when solving word problems or equations. Table 5.8 presents the formula, what each component of the formula means, and a graphic representation. You should be familiar with these formulas.

Table 5.8
Formulas

Name	Formula	Graphic
Area (A) of a circle	$A = \pi r^2$, where $\pi = 3.14$ and r = radius	
Area (A) of a parallelogram	$A = bh$, where b = base and h = height	
Area (A) of a rectangle	$A = lw$, where l = length and w = width	
Area (A) of a square	$A = s^2$, where s = side	
Area (A) of a trapezoid	$A = \frac{1}{2} h\,(b + a)$, where h = height, a = lower base, and b = upper base	
Area (A) of a triangle	$A = \frac{1}{2} bh$, where b = base and h = height	

Table 5.8
Formulas

Name	Formula	Graphic
Circumference (C) of a circle	$C = \pi d$, where $\pi = 3.14$ and d = diameter	
Distance (D)	$D = rt$, where r = rate and t = time	
Mean (Average)	$\text{Average} = \dfrac{\text{Sum of the } n \text{ values}}{N}$ where Sum of the n values = all of the numbers in the set added together and N = the total of numbers in the set	
Percent Change (PC)	$PC = \dfrac{\text{Amount of change}}{\text{Original cost}}$	
Perimeter (P) of a parallelogram	$P = 2l + 2w$, where l = length and w = width	
Perimeter (P) of a rectangle	$P = 2l + 2w$, where l = length and w = width	
Perimeter (P) of a square	$P = 4s$, where s = side	
Perimeter (P) of a triangle	$P = a + b + c$, where a, b, and c are the sides	

Table 5.8
Formulas

Name	Formula	Graphic
Perimeter (P) of a trapezoid	$P = b_1 + b_2 + s_1 + s_2$, where b_1 = lower base, b_2 = upper base, s_1 = one side, and s_2 = the opposite side	
Probability (P)	$P = \dfrac{\text{Number of successful outcomes}}{\text{Number of possible outcomes}}$	
Pythagorean Theorem	$c^2 = a^2 + b^2$, where $c =$ hypotenuse and a and b are legs of a right triangle	
Ratio and proportion	$A = B :: C = D$ or $\dfrac{A}{B} = \dfrac{C}{D} = (AD)(BC)$, where one side of the equation, either A and B or C and D is known and only one component of the remaining equation is known	
Selling price (SP)	$SP = c + o + p$, where c = cost, o = overhead, and p = profit	
Simple interest (I)	$I = P \times R \times T$, where P = principal, R = rate, and T = time	
Surface Area (SA) of a cube	$SA = s \times s \times 6$, where s = length of a side	

Table 5.8
Formulas

Name	Formula	Graphic
Surface Area (*SA*) of a cylinder	$SA = 2(\pi r^2) + h(2\pi r)$	
Surface Area (*SA*) of a rectangular solid	$A = 2lw + 2wh + 2lh$, where *lw* = area of bottom and top, *wh* = area of sides, and *lh* = area of back and front	
Volume (*V*) of cube	$V = s \times s \times s$, where *s* = length of a side	
Volume (*V*) of cylinder	$V = \pi r^2 \times h$, where $\pi = 3.14$, *r* = radius, and *h* = height	
Volume (*V*) of rectangular solid	$V = l \times w \times h$, where *l* = length, *w* = width, and *h* = height	

Answer Sheet
SAMPLE TEST

Algebra

1 Ⓐ Ⓑ Ⓒ Ⓓ   10 Ⓐ Ⓑ Ⓒ Ⓓ   19 Ⓐ Ⓑ Ⓒ Ⓓ
2 Ⓐ Ⓑ Ⓒ Ⓓ   11 Ⓐ Ⓑ Ⓒ Ⓓ   20 Ⓐ Ⓑ Ⓒ Ⓓ
3 Ⓐ Ⓑ Ⓒ Ⓓ   12 Ⓐ Ⓑ Ⓒ Ⓓ   21 Ⓐ Ⓑ Ⓒ Ⓓ
4 Ⓐ Ⓑ Ⓒ Ⓓ   13 Ⓐ Ⓑ Ⓒ Ⓓ   22 Ⓐ Ⓑ Ⓒ Ⓓ
5 Ⓐ Ⓑ Ⓒ Ⓓ   14 Ⓐ Ⓑ Ⓒ Ⓓ   23 Ⓐ Ⓑ Ⓒ Ⓓ
6 Ⓐ Ⓑ Ⓒ Ⓓ   15 Ⓐ Ⓑ Ⓒ Ⓓ   24 Ⓐ Ⓑ Ⓒ Ⓓ
7 Ⓐ Ⓑ Ⓒ Ⓓ   16 Ⓐ Ⓑ Ⓒ Ⓓ   25 Ⓐ Ⓑ Ⓒ Ⓓ
8 Ⓐ Ⓑ Ⓒ Ⓓ   17 Ⓐ Ⓑ Ⓒ Ⓓ
9 Ⓐ Ⓑ Ⓒ Ⓓ   18 Ⓐ Ⓑ Ⓒ Ⓓ

Algebra Sample Test

Algebra Sample Test

Directions: For each question, select the letter (A, B, C, or D) that corresponds with your answer. Record your answers on the answer sheet on page 147.

1. If $5x - 6 = 24$, then $x + 5 =$

   (A) 11
   (B) 7
   (C) 15
   (D) 12

2. If $x + 7x - 16 = 0$, then $x =$

   (A) 2.29
   (B) 3
   (C) 2
   (D) 4

3. If $7(b + 7) - 5b - 13 = 0$, then $3b =$ **CHALLENGE**

   (A) 13
   (B) –15
   (C) –54
   (D) 31

4. If $\dfrac{1}{6}x + \dfrac{1}{5}x + \dfrac{3}{10}x = 90$, then $x =$

   (A) 60
   (B) 85
   (C) 105
   (D) 135

5. Solve for a in the proportion: a is to 10 as 6 is to 20.

   (A) 12
   (B) 20
   (C) 3
   (D) 6

6. If $3(5 \cdot 2) = 6(x + 3)$, then $x =$

   (A) 1.66
   (B) 2
   (C) 8
   (D) 4

7. Evaluate $x^3 - x^2 + 15$ if $x = 2$

   (A) 19   **CHALLENGE**
   (B) 15
   (C) 0
   (D) 10

8. If $15 - x = 13$, then $x =$

   (A) 28
   (B) 2
   (C) –2
   (D) 14

9. If $5x + 6 = 3x$, then $x =$

   (A) 0.75
   (B) 3.6
   (C) –3
   (D) 0.10

10. If $\dfrac{4}{5}x = 50$, then $x =$

    (A) 40
    (B) 400
    (C) 10
    (D) 62.5

11. Solve $\dfrac{x + y}{5} + 5x - 3y$ if $x = 8$ and $y = 10$

    (A) 29
    (B) 26
    (C) 73.3
    (D) 13.6

12. Solve for x in the proportion: 15 is to 80 as x is to 10

    (A) 53.33
    (B) 1.875
    (C) 120
    (D) 64

Algebra Sample Test

13. If $8x - 7 = 3x + 10$, then $x =$
   (A) 3.4
   (B) 0.6
   (C) 27.2
   (D) 6

14. If $x + 15 = 95$, then $x =$
   (A) 110
   (B) −15
   (C) 80
   (D) 40

15. If $\frac{3}{4}b + 15 = 50$, then $b =$
   (A) 2.92
   (B) 46.7
   (C) 65
   (D) 35

16. If $\frac{b}{5} = \frac{7}{1}$, then $b =$
   (A) 35
   (B) 5
   (C) 40
   (D) 12

17. If $(4x + 7) \div 5 = 58$, then $x =$
   (A) 12.75
   (B) 1.15
   (C) 74.25
   (D) 70.75

18. Evaluate $5ab^2 + 3(a^2 + b^3)$ when $a = 4$ and $b = 7$.

   CHALLENGE

   (A) 1,175
   (B) 1,400
   (C) 2,057
   (D) 1,682

19. If $4x + 3(7x + 15) = 195$, then $x =$
   (A) 5
   (B) 6
   (C) 7.5
   (D) 8.4

20. If $5a - 10 = 3a + 4$, then $a =$
   (A) −0.75
   (B) 7
   (C) 3
   (D) 4.5

21. If $\frac{2}{3}x + \frac{4}{5}(x - 5)$, then $x =$
   (A) 57.3
   (B) 51.82
   (C) 6.36
   (D) 2.97

22. If $8x - 17 = 425$, then $x =$
   (A) 62.74
   (B) 51
   (C) 47.89
   (D) 55.25

23. If $8 + 4(x - 15) = 42$, then $x =$
   (A) −2.5
   (B) 23.5
   (C) 25.5
   (D) 12.5

24. If $(7b + 3) \div 3 = 80$, then $2b =$
   (A) 67.72
   (B) 22.86
   (C) 38.86
   (D) 45.71

25. If $\frac{3}{7} = \frac{b}{15}$, then $b =$
   (A) 1.4
   (B) 6.43
   (C) 35
   (D) 7

Algebra Sample Test Answer Key

1. **(A)** $5x - 6 = 24$
$5x = 30$
$x = 6$
$6 + 5 = 11$

2. **(C)** $x + 7x - 16 = 0$
$8x - 16 = 0$
$8x = 16$
$x = 2$

3. **(C)** $7(b + 7) - 5b - 13 = 0$
$7b + 49 - 5b - 13 = 0$
$2b + 36 = 0$
$2b = -36$
$b = -18$
$3(-18) = -54$

4. **(D)** $\dfrac{1}{6}x + \dfrac{1}{5}x + \dfrac{3}{10}x = 90$
$\dfrac{5}{30}x + \dfrac{6}{30}x + \dfrac{9}{30}x = 90$
$\dfrac{20}{30}x = 90$
$x = 135$

5. **(C)** $a : 10 = 6 : 20$
$(a)(20) = (10)(6)$
$20a = 60$
$a = 3$

6. **(B)** $3(5 \cdot 2) = 6(x + 3)$
$3(10) = 6x + 18$
$30 = 6x + 18$
$12 = 6x$
$2 = x$

7. **(A)** $x^3 - x^2 + 15 = (2 \cdot 2 \cdot 2) - (2 \cdot 2) + 15$
$= 8 - 4 + 15 = 19$

8. **(B)** $15 - x = 13$
$x = 2$

9. **(C)** $5x + 6 = 3x$
$2x + 6 = 0$
$2x = -6$
$x = -3$

10. **(D)** $\dfrac{4}{5}x = 50$
$x = 62.5$

11. **(D)** $\dfrac{x + y}{5} + 5x - 3y =$
$\dfrac{8 + 10}{5} + 5(8) - 3(10) =$
$\dfrac{18}{5} + 40 - 30 =$
$3.6 + 40 - 30 = 13.6$

12. **(B)** $15 : 80 = x : 10$
$(80)(x) = (15)(10)$
$80x = 150$
$x = 1.875$

13. **(A)** $8x - 7 = 3x + 10$
$5x - 7 = 10$
$5x = 17$
$x = 3.4$

14. **(C)** $x + 15 = 95$
$x = 80$

15. **(B)** $\dfrac{3}{4}b + 15 = 50$
$\dfrac{3}{4}b = 35$
$b = 46.7$

16. **(A)** $\dfrac{b}{5} = 7$
$b = 35$

17. **(D)** $\dfrac{4x + 7}{5} = 58$
$4x + 7 = 290$
$4x = 283$
$x = 70.75$

18. **(C)** $5ab^2 + 3(a^2 + b^3) =$
$5(4)(7^2) + 3(4^2 + 7^3) =$
$5(4)(49) + 3(16 + 343) =$
$980 + 1,077 = 2,057$

19. **(B)** $4x + 3(7x + 15) = 195$
$4x + 21x + 45 = 195$
$25x + 45 = 195$
$25x = 150$
$x = 6$

20. **(B)** $5a - 10 = 3a + 4$
$5a = 3a + 14$
$2a = 14$
$a = 7$

21. **(A)** $\frac{2}{3}x + \frac{4}{5}(x - 5) = 80$
$10x + 12(x - 5) = 1,200$
$10x + 12x - 60 = 1,200$
$22x = 1,260$
$x = 57.3$

22. **(D)** $8x - 17 = 425$
$8x = 442$
$x = 55.25$

23. **(B)** $8 + 4(x - 15) = 42$
$8 + 4x - 60 = 42$
$4x - 52 = 42$
$4x = 94$
$x = 23.5$

24. **(A)** $\frac{7b + 3}{3} = 80$
$7b + 3 = 240$
$7b = 237$
$b = 33.86$
$2b = 67.72$

25. **(B)** $\frac{3}{7} = \frac{b}{15}$
$7b = 45$
$b = 6.43$

Geometry Review

Geometry is the study of shapes and figures in either two or three dimensions. Plane geometry studies shapes and figures in two dimensions, whereas solid geometry studies shapes and figures in three dimensions.

Lines and Points

In geometry the word *line* always indicates a straight line. A line extends indefinitely in one or two directions. Straight lines are actually composed of an indefinite number of points. The following illustration is a line with three points. An arrow or arrows at one or both ends of the line indicate the direction of the line.

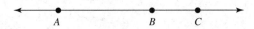

The line is *AC* and is written $\overleftrightarrow{AC}$. Lines may also be identified by using an italicized lowercase letter as in the following illustration. When identified in lowercase one or two directional arrows are used.

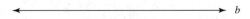

Since lines are made up of infinite points, it is possible to identify a portion or part of a line. This identified part of a line is called a *line segment*. Such segments are identified in one of two formats. A line without arrows may be drawn above the letters identifying the segment, or simply the letters without a line may indicate the line segment. In the following illustration, *AB*, *BC*, and *CD* are line segments of the line *AD*.

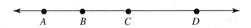

A *ray*, unlike a straight line, has a definite endpoint and proceeds only in one direction. A ray is identified by the letter placed at the end point or any other point on the ray. The symbol placed above the letter identifying the ray indicates the direction of the ray. The ray illustrated here is written $\overrightarrow{GH}$.

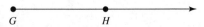

Lines are more than just single entities. There are a number of ways in which lines can be presented. *Intersecting lines* are just what the words indicate—the lines intersect or cross each other. In the next diagram the lines $\overleftrightarrow{AB}$ and $\overleftrightarrow{CD}$ intersect at *Y*.

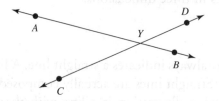

Perpendicular lines also intersect, but as opposed to intersecting lines, perpendicular lines always form 90° angles where they intersect.

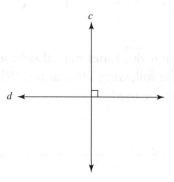

The small box (□) where lines *c* and *d* intersect denotes a 90° angle. The box is used with diagrams. When writing about perpendicular lines, the symbol ⊥ is used.

A third type of line are the parallel lines. *Parallel lines* do not intersect but continue with a constant, unchanging distance between them. Lines *s* and *t* in the following diagram are parallel lines.

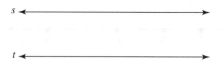

Parallel lines may be intersected or crossed by another or *transverse line.* With transverse lines, both parallel lines must be crossed by a straight line. In the following diagram, the line *z* crosses the parallel lines *s* and *t*.

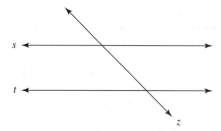

Geometric Figures

Shapes and figures used in geometry determine the type of geometry present. As mentioned earlier, plane geometry is two dimensional and is represented by flat figures. Solid geometry is represented by figures that have three dimensions or shape. We live in a three-dimensional world.

Angles

Angles are two rays that have a common endpoint. An angle has two components, the vertex or point where the two endpoints meet, and the sides of the angle or the rays. Angles are labeled according to their vertex and endpoints, their vertex, or by a numeral or lowercase letter inside the angle. Angles are measured in degrees from 0° to 360°.

SINGLE ANGLE TYPES

There are a number of types of single angles. You should be able to identify an angle by looking at it. The angle in the next diagram is a *right* angle. Such angles have a measurement of 90°. Angles with more or less than 90° are not right angles. The right angle could be labeled ∠*A*, ∠*CAB*, or ∠*BAC*.

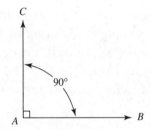

The following angle is an *acute* angle. Such angles have a measure of less than 90°. This acute angle could be labeled ∠*E*, ∠1, ∠*DEF*, or ∠*FED*.

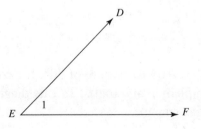

Obtuse angles are angles measuring more than 90° but less than 180°. The following obtuse angle could be labeled $\angle T$, $\angle RTS$, $\angle 2$, or $\angle STR$.

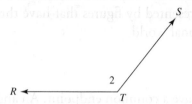

The last type of angle is the *straight* angle. A straight angle has a measure of 180°. If the angle has more or less than 180° it is not a straight angle. The following straight angle is labeled $\angle ACE$ or $\angle ECA$.

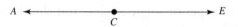

MULTIPLE ANGLE TYPES

Angles may occur with other angles. Just as there are different types of single angles, there are different types of multiple angles. *Adjacent* angles share a common side or ray and have the same vertex or meeting point. In the next diagram, $\overleftrightarrow{AC}$ is the common side of the two angles, and $\angle A$ is the vertex. The diagram indicates that $\angle 1$ and $\angle 2$ are adjacent angles, as are angles $\angle BAC$ and $\angle CAD$.

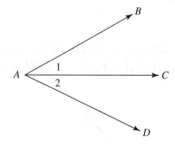

Complementary angles have a total measure of 90°. If two angles are more or less than 90°, they are not complementary angles. In this diagram, $\angle 1 + \angle 2 = 90°$, as does $\angle ABC$ since it is a right triangle.

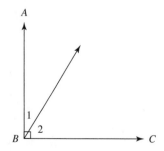

Perpendicular angles are formed when two lines intersect and form right triangles at their common vertex. In the following diagram, ∠1, ∠2, ∠3, and ∠4 each measure 90°. The sum of the four angles is 360°. Each angle is also a right triangle.

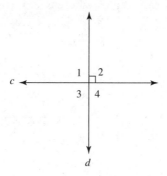

Supplementary angles are two angles whose measure equals 180°. Two angles with a measure of more or less than 180° are not supplementary. In this diagram, ∠1 + ∠2 = 180°. Supplementary angles always form a straight line.

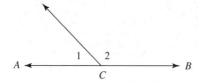

Vertical angles are formed when two lines intersect but do not form 90° angles at their common vertex or meeting point. In vertical angles, opposite angles have equal measures. In the following diagram ∠1 and ∠3 have equal measures, as do ∠2 and ∠4. Also, ∠1 and ∠2, ∠2 and ∠3, ∠3 and ∠4, and ∠4 and ∠1 each measure 180°. The sum of the four measures, that is, ∠1 through ∠4, is 360°. Also note that *AB* and *CD* are lines with measures of 180° each.

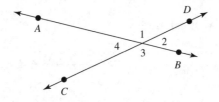

Interior and *exterior* angles are formed when a transversal line intersects with two parallel lines. Interior angles are those angles on the inside of the parallel lines. Exterior angles are those angles outside of the parallel lines. In the next diagram, $\angle 1$, $\angle 2$, $\angle 7$, and $\angle 8$ are exterior angles whereas $\angle 3$, $\angle 4$, $\angle 5$, and $\angle 6$ are interior angles.

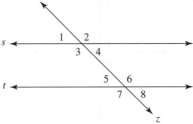

This intersection of one line with two parallel lines forms a number of relationships worth remembering.

1. $\angle 1$, $\angle 2$, $\angle 3$, and $\angle 4$ are identical to $\angle 5$, $\angle 6$, $\angle 7$, and $\angle 8$. In this case, the following angles are identical or corresponding angles:

   $\angle 1 = \angle 5$ $\qquad\qquad\qquad$ $\angle 2 = \angle 6$

   $\angle 3 = \angle 7$ $\qquad\qquad\qquad$ $\angle 4 = \angle 8$

2. The following angles are both adjacent and supplementary angles:

   $\angle 1 + \angle 3 = 180°$ $\qquad\qquad$ $\angle 2 + \angle 4 = 180°$

   $\angle 5 + \angle 7 = 180°$ $\qquad\qquad$ $\angle 6 + \angle 8 = 180°$

   $\angle 1 + \angle 2 = 180°$ $\qquad\qquad$ $\angle 3 + \angle 4 = 180°$

   $\angle 5 + \angle 6 = 180°$ $\qquad\qquad$ $\angle 7 + \angle 8 = 180°$

3. The following are vertical angles:

   $\angle 1$ and $\angle 4$ $\qquad\qquad\qquad$ $\angle 2$ and $\angle 3$

   $\angle 5$ and $\angle 8$ $\qquad\qquad\qquad$ $\angle 6$ and $\angle 7$

4. If the measure of one of the eight angles is known, the measures of the remaining angles can be determined.

EXAMPLE 1

Using the preceding diagram, assume that $\angle 5 = 45°$. Determine the measures of the remaining angles. There are a number of different approaches to solving the problem. One approach follows:

a. $\angle 5$ and $\angle 6$ are located on line t, which has a total measure of 180°. Subtract the measure of $\angle 5$ from 180° to determine the measure of $\angle 6$.

$$180° - 45° = 135° = \angle 6$$

b. The angles on line s and line t are identical, so if $\angle 5 = 45°$, then $\angle 1 = 45°$, and if $\angle 6 = 135°$, then $\angle 2 = 135°$.

c. $\angle 1$ and $\angle 4$, and $\angle 5$ and $\angle 8$ are vertical angles and are, therefore, equal in measurement. If $\angle 1$ and $\angle 5$ are each equal to 45°, then $\angle 4$ and $\angle 8$ are also 45° each.

d. $\angle 2$ and $\angle 3$, and $\angle 6$ and $\angle 8$ are vertical angles and are equal in measurement. If $\angle 2$ and $\angle 6$ are 135° each, then $\angle 3$ and $\angle 7$ are also 135° each.

e. The answer to the problem is if $\angle 5 = 45°$, then

$\angle 1 = 45°$	$\angle 2 = 135°$
$\angle 3 = 135°$	$\angle 4 = 45°$
$\angle 6 = 135°$	$\angle 7 = 135°$
$\angle 8 = 45°$	

Circles

Circles, as opposed to lines, come about and join together. They do not extend into space for an indefinite distance. Like the line, the circle is composed of an infinite number of points, but the points in a circle are all equidistant from an imaginary or identified point in the center of the circle. The center of the circle is labeled with an uppercase letter, as are the points around the circle.

A circle has three parts, the circumference (c) or distance around the circle, the diameter (d) or distance across the circle going through the center point, and the radius (r) or half the distance of the diameter going from a point on the circle to its center point.

The area and circumference of a circle can be determined. Refer to Table 5.8 for specific formulas and graphic representations for circular objects.

Polygons

Polygons are closed two-dimensional shapes or figures having three or more sides. Two-dimensional objects are flat objects. Triangles, squares, rectangles, octagons, and hexagons are all examples of polygons.

TRIANGLES

Figures or shapes having three sides are triangles. Triangles have three interior angles that total 180°. A figure or shape measuring more or less than 180° is not a triangle.

There are many types of triangles. Triangles are classified according to their shape or by their angles. Triangles are classified according to their shape:

- Isosceles triangles *have two equal sides and, therefore, two equal angles plus an additional angle.*

- Equilateral triangles *have three sides equal, and each of the three angles is equal to 60°.*

- Scalene triangles *have no equal sides or angles.*

Triangles are also classified by their angles:

- Acute triangles *have each interior angle or measure less than 90°.*

- Obtuse triangles *have one interior angle or measure greater than 90° but less than 180°.*

- Right triangles *have one interior angle or measure of 90°.*

SQUARES AND RECTANGLES

Two-dimensional shapes or figures with four sides are squares or rectangles. The total measurement for a square or rectangle is 360°. Both squares and rectangles have four sides with each angle equal to 90°. Squares and rectangles are composed of right angles.

Squares and rectangles differ in the length of their sides. Squares have four sides of equal length, whereas rectangles have two sides of one length and two sides of another length. The equal sides are opposite each other in the rectangle.

The area, or the measure within the figure, and perimeter, or distance around the figure, can be determined for triangles, squares, and rectangles. See Table 5.8 for the formulas for finding the area of various polygons and their graphic representations.

Pythagorean Theorem

The Pythagorean Theorem applies to right triangles only. It states that the sum of the squares of two legs of the triangle is equal to the square of the hypotenuse or third leg. The theorem is employed when working with right triangles when two of the three sides are known, and the third side is unknown. In most instances, the theorem is used for indirect measurement when it is impractical or impossible to measure directly. Refer to Table 5.8 for the formula and graphic representation of the Pythagorean Theorem.

Cubes, Rectangular Solids, and Cylinders

Cubes, rectangular solids, and cylinders are three-dimensional objects. They might be thought of as extensions of the square, rectangle, and circle. For three-dimensional figures, volume is expressed in terms of *cubic* inches, centimeters, or feet. The volume, or amount of space within the object, and surface area, the outer area of the object, of cubes, rectangular solids, and cylinders can be mathematically determined. Refer to Table 5.8 for exact formulas and graphic representations of each three-dimensional object.

Answer Sheet
SAMPLE TEST

Geometry

1 Ⓐ Ⓑ Ⓒ Ⓓ   10 Ⓐ Ⓑ Ⓒ Ⓓ   19 Ⓐ Ⓑ Ⓒ Ⓓ
2 Ⓐ Ⓑ Ⓒ Ⓓ   11 Ⓐ Ⓑ Ⓒ Ⓓ   20 Ⓐ Ⓑ Ⓒ Ⓓ
3 Ⓐ Ⓑ Ⓒ Ⓓ   12 Ⓐ Ⓑ Ⓒ Ⓓ   21 Ⓐ Ⓑ Ⓒ Ⓓ
4 Ⓐ Ⓑ Ⓒ Ⓓ   13 Ⓐ Ⓑ Ⓒ Ⓓ   22 Ⓐ Ⓑ Ⓒ Ⓓ
5 Ⓐ Ⓑ Ⓒ Ⓓ   14 Ⓐ Ⓑ Ⓒ Ⓓ   23 Ⓐ Ⓑ Ⓒ Ⓓ
6 Ⓐ Ⓑ Ⓒ Ⓓ   15 Ⓐ Ⓑ Ⓒ Ⓓ   24 Ⓐ Ⓑ Ⓒ Ⓓ
7 Ⓐ Ⓑ Ⓒ Ⓓ   16 Ⓐ Ⓑ Ⓒ Ⓓ   25 Ⓐ Ⓑ Ⓒ Ⓓ
8 Ⓐ Ⓑ Ⓒ Ⓓ   17 Ⓐ Ⓑ Ⓒ Ⓓ
9 Ⓐ Ⓑ Ⓒ Ⓓ   18 Ⓐ Ⓑ Ⓒ Ⓓ

Geometry Sample Test

Directions: For each question, select the letter (A, B, C, or D) that corresponds with your answer. Record your answers on the answer sheet on page 163.

Questions 1–3 refer to the following diagram.

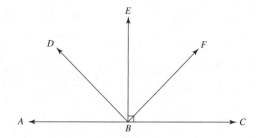

1. The number of degrees in ∠*EBA* is

    (A) 80°.
    (B) 90°.
    (C) 140°.
    (D) 180°.

2. _____ is an acute angle.

    (A) ∠*DBC*
    (B) ∠*ABC*
    (C) ∠*ABE*
    (D) ∠*DBA*

3. If ∠*EBC* is 90°, then ∠*FBC* is

    (A) 90°.
    (B) 45°.
    (C) 15°.
    (D) 5°.

4. The diameter of a circle is 50 inches. The radius of the circle is

    (A) 100 inches.
    (B) 25 inches.
    (C) 157 inches.
    (D) 45 inches.

5. If two angles of a triangle have a total measure of 95°, the third angle has a measure of

    (A) 180°.
    (B) 265°.
    (C) 90°.
    (D) 85°.

6. An obtuse angle has a measure of

    (A) less than 90° but larger than 45°.
    (B) more than 90° but less than 180°.
    (C) equal to 90° but less than 360°.
    (D) 180°.

7. In the following diagram, ∠*ABC* is a right triangle. The ∠*ABD* has a measure of 50° and ∠*DBC* has a measure of 40°. The two angles are called

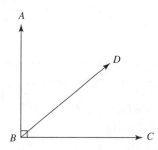

    (A) supplementary angles.
    (B) supporting angles.
    (C) complementary angles.
    (D) pairs of angles.

8. The following diagram is a _____ triangle.

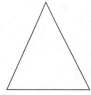

    (A) scalene
    (B) isosceles
    (C) concave
    (D) right

9. If, in the following diagram, ∠*ABE* has a measure of 130°, then ∠*y* has a measure of

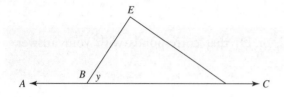

(A) 50°.
(B) y^2.
(C) 230°.
(D) Not enough information is given to make a determination.

10. Determine *x* for a right triangle where the hypotenuse is equal to 5 and one leg is equal to 4.

(A) 9
(B) 3
(C) 1
(D) 5

CHALLENGE

11. A circle has a radius of 7 inches. Determine the circumference of the circle.

(A) 21.98 inches
(B) 153.86 inches
(C) 138.03 inches
(D) 43.96 inches

12. Determine the volume of the following rectangular solid.

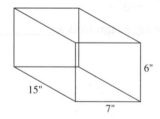

(A) 99 cubic inches
(B) 99 inches
(C) 630 cubic inches
(D) 630 inches

13. Determine the perimeter of the following triangle.

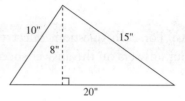

(A) 27″
(B) 53″
(C) 43″
(D) 45″

14. Determine the area of the following trapezoid.

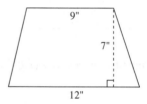

(A) 28 square inches
(B) 73.5 square inches
(C) 756 square inches
(D) 14.3 square inches

15. Determine the area of a circle whose diameter is 8 inches.

(A) 50.24 square inches
(B) 50.24 inches
(C) 200.96 square inches
(D) 200.96 inches

16. If three angles of a square measure 270°, what is the measure of the fourth angle?

(A) 90°
(B) 180°
(C) 300°
(D) 30°

17. Determine *x* in the following right triangle.

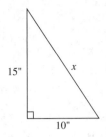

(A) 25″
(B) 18″
(C) 32.5″
(D) 20″

18. Determine the area of the following parallelogram.

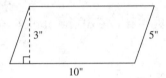

(A) 18 square inches
(B) 35 square inches
(C) 30 square inches
(D) 25 square inches

19. Determine the volume of a cube whose sides are each 13″.

(A) 169 cubic inches
(B) 52 cubic inches
(C) 109.8 cubic inches
(D) 2,197 cubic inches

CHALLENGE

20. A quadrilateral figure has how many sides?

(A) 3
(B) 4
(C) 5
(D) 6

21. The perimeter of a square is 40 inches. Determine the area of the square.

(A) 160 square inches
(B) 10 square inches
(C) 100 square inches
(D) 80 square inches

22. Determine the perimeter of the following figure.

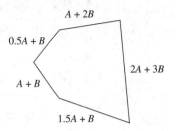

(A) $A^2 + B^2$
(B) $0.5(A^2 + B^2)$
(C) $5(6A + 9B)$
(D) $6A + 8B$

23. Which object has the greater volume?

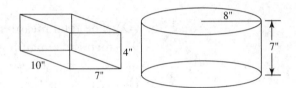

(A) The volume of the cylinder with 1,406.72 cubic inches is greater.
(B) The volume of the rectangular solid with 280 cubic inches is greater.
(C) They will hold equal amounts.
(D) Rectangular solids and cylinders can't be compared because of the difference in shapes.

CHALLENGE

24. Does the circle or the triangle contain the greatest measure of degrees?

(A) The circle
(B) The triangle
(C) Both contain the same measure of degree since both are two-dimensional figures.
(D) There is not enough information given to determine an answer.

25. $\triangle ABC$ is a right isosceles triangle. If $\angle A = \angle C$, then $\angle B =$

(A) 90°
(B) 35°
(C) 30°
(D) 45°

CHALLENGE

Geometry Sample Test Answer Key

1. **(B)** $\angle EBA$ is a right angle.

2. **(D)** An acute angle is less than 90°.

3. **(B)** One half of a right angle has a measure of 45°.

4. **(B)** The radius of a circle is one half of the diameter.

   $d = 50''$

   $r = \dfrac{1}{2}d$

   $r = \dfrac{1}{2}(50'')$

   $r = 25''$

5. **(D)** The total measure of a triangle is 180°. If two of the angles are equal to 95° then the remaining angle is 85°.

6. **(B)** Obtuse angles are more than 90° but less than 180°.

7. **(C)** Complementary angles have a total measure of 90°.

8. **(B)** Isosceles triangles have 2 equal sides or angles.

9. **(A)** A straight angle has a measure of 180°. $\overleftrightarrow{AC}$ is a straight angle. If $\angle ABE = 130°$, then $\angle y = 50°$.

10. **(B)** Let side $a = x$, $b = 4$, and $c = 5$.

    $a^2 + b^2 = c^2$

    $a^2 + 4^2 = 5^2$

    $a^2 + 16 = 25$

    $a^2 = 9$

    $a = \sqrt{9}$

    $a = 3 = x$

11. **(D)** $d = 2r = 2 \times 7 = 14''$

    $C = \pi d$

    $C = (3.14)(14)$

    $C = 43.96''$

12. **(C)** $V = lwh$

    $V = (15)(7)(6)$

    $V = 630$ cubic inches

13. **(D)** $P = s_1 + s_2 + s_3$
$P = 10'' + 15'' + 20''$
$P = 45''$

14. **(B)** $A = \dfrac{1}{2}(b_1 + b_2)h$

$A = \dfrac{1}{2}(9'' + 12'')7''$

$A = \dfrac{1}{2}(21'')7''$

$A = 73.5$ square inches

15. **(A)** $r = \dfrac{1}{2}d = \dfrac{1}{2}(8 \text{ inches}) = 4 \text{ inches}$

$A = \pi r^2$
$A = (3.14)(4 \text{ inches})^2$
$A = (3.14)(16 \text{ square inches})$
$A = 50.24$ square inches

16. **(A)** A square has four equal sides and four equal angles of 90° each, or a total measure of 360°. If a square has three angles measuring 270°, then the remaining angle has a measure of 90°.

17. **(B)** $a^2 + b^2 = c^2$
$10^2 + 15^2 = c^2$
$100 + 225 = c^2$
$325 = c^2$
$\sqrt{325} = c$
$18 \text{ inches} = c$

18. **(C)** $A = bh$
$A = (10 \text{ inches})(3 \text{ inches})$
$A = 30$ square inches

19. **(D)** $V = s^3$
$V = (13'')^3$
$V = (13'')(13'')(13'')$
$V = 2{,}197$ cubic inches

20. **(B)** Quadrilaterals have four sides.

21. **(C)** $A = s^2$
$A = 10^2$
$A = (10)(10)$
$A = 100$

22. **(D)** $(A + 2B) + (2A + 3B) + (1.5A + B) + (A + B) + (0.5A + B) = 6A + 8B$

23. **(A) Volume of rectangular solid**
    $V = lwh$
    $V = $ (4 inches)(7 inches)(10 inches)
    $V = 280$ cubic inches

    Volume of cylinder
    $V = \pi r^2 h$
    $V = $ (3.14)(8 inches)^2(7 inches)
    $V = $ (3.14)(64 square inches)(7 inches)
    $V = 1,406.72$ cubic inches

24. **(A)** A circle contains 360°, whereas a triangle contains 180°.

25. **(A)** Right isosceles triangles have one angle with a measure of 90°, and the two remaining angles are equal.
    $$\angle A = x$$
    $$\angle C = x$$
    $$x + x + 90° = 180°$$
    $$2x + 90° = 180°$$
    $$2x = 90°$$
    $$x = 45°$$

Verbal Problem Review

Verbal problems mirror events or problems encountered in life, and like problems encountered in life, verbal problems can be difficult to solve if you are not sure of what you are doing, get in a hurry, or leave out a step.

Verbal problems can address any life event and can use any type of mathematics. A verbal problem may ask about the interest rate on a loan, how to find the average grade for a course, or how much medication to give a patient. The problem may ask about distance traveled or how far a group of hikers is from their home base after they changed directions and walked a set distance.

With regard to mathematics, a verbal problem may ask for nothing more than simple arithmetic, or it may include several steps and use principles of algebra and geometry. Verbal problems may require specific formulas or units of measurement in order to solve the problem. It's important to go beyond mere memorization of formulas. Know when to use the formula and how to apply it correctly. Learn both English as well as metric units of measurement. See Table 5.8 for specific formulas to use with verbal problems.

When solving verbal problems, take your time, read carefully, and do not become overly anxious if you think you cannot solve the problem. Work the problem one step at a time, and do not try to jump ahead or jump to an answer. Consider the following when working verbal problems:

1. What is the problem asking you to do? If you can write in your test booklet or on your exam, underline or circle what you need to know.

2. What information does the problem give you? The problem must give you a certain amount of information in order for you to solve the problem. Mark this information on your exam if possible. Does the problem give you information in yards and then ask for the answer in inches?

3. Make a simple diagram or sketch of the information the problem gives you and use an X or a question mark to indicate what you need to find out. Label what you know. Some verbal problems may give you more information than what you need, so pay attention to what the problem is asking you to do. Do not waste time trying to make the perfect sketch, but make it good enough so that you understand what you mean.

4. Look for conversions you might need to make before you solve the problem. Do you need to go from ounces to pounds or from the English system to the metric system. Remember that you will not get the correct answer if you are trying to compare feet and inches or milliliters and teaspoons.

5. Consider the expressions or equations you might use to solve the problem. Is there a specific formula that you can use to answer the question the verbal problem poses? If there is a formula, determine which components of the formula are defined. If there is not a specific formula, how will you set up the problem to solve it?

6. Solve the equation or expression. Add, subtract, multiply, and divide carefully. Many errors are caused by a lack of focus or hurrying. Double-check how you worked the problem. If your answers do not agree, look for simple mistakes like $2 + 2 = 5$, $3 \times 3 = 6$, or $30 - 25 = 55$.

7. Look at your answer and then look at what the question asked. Is your answer sensible? Have you answered the question posed in the verbal problem? The majority of verbal problems are based on events occurring in everyday life, so it's doubtful that you would get an answer suggesting a man could run 100 miles per hour.

Age Problems

EXAMPLE 1

Sally and John are brother and sister. Sally is 5 years older than John. Sally was born on their father's 22nd birthday in 1965. In what year was John born?

x = the year that Sally was born or the year 1965

$x + 5$ = the year that John was born since he was born 5 years after Sally was born

$x + 5 = 1965 + 5 = 1970$ = the year of John's birth

The age of Sally and John's father has nothing to do with the problem.

EXAMPLE 2

Martin and Mary are brother and sister. Martin is two times as old as Mary. There is 27 years between their ages. How old are Martin and Mary?

x = Mary's age

$2x$ = Martin's age since he is twice Mary's age

27 = difference in years between Mary and Martin

$2x - x = 27$

$x = 27$

Mary's age = x = 27

Martin's age = $2x$ = 54

Distance Problems

EXAMPLE 1

Two trains leave from two different cities that are 650 miles apart. They are traveling toward each other. The Prairie Flyer averages 72 miles per hour. The Mountain Breeze averages 55 miles per hour. Both trains left their respective stations at the same time. How many hours will it take for the two trains to meet?

T = the number of hours it will take for the two trains to meet

R = 72 = the average speed of the Prairie Flyer

R = 55 = the average speed of the Mountain Breeze

650 = the total distance to be covered by both trains

Distance = (Rate)(Time) or $D = RT$

$R \cdot T = D$

$72T + 55T = 650$

$127T = 650$

$T = 5.118$ or 5.12 hours

EXAMPLE 2

Two long-distance runners are 50 miles apart. They start running toward each other at 7:00 A.M. Runner One runs an average 4 miles per hour, and Runner Two runs an average of 1.5 miles per ten minutes. What time will the runners meet?

T = the time it takes the two runners to cover 50 miles

R = 4 = the average number of miles run per hour by Runner One

R = 9 = the average number of miles run per hour by Runner Two

50 = the total distance covered by both runners

1.5 miles : 10 minutes = x miles : 60 minutes

$$10x = 90$$

$$x = 9 \text{ miles}$$

$R \cdot T = D$

$4T + 9T = 50$

$13T = 50$

$T = 3.8$ hours or 3 hours 48 minutes

The two runners will meet at 10:48 A.M.

Ratio and Proportion Problems

EXAMPLE 1

A cake recipe and its cooked icing call for a total of 11 eggs. You plan to bake 3 cakes with icing for the charity bazaar. How many dozen eggs will you have to buy to bake the 3 cakes and make the icing for each?

$$1 \text{ recipe} : 11 \text{ eggs} = 3 \text{ recipes} : x \text{ eggs}$$

$$33 \text{ eggs} = x$$

$$1 \text{ dozen eggs} : 12 \text{ eggs} = x \text{ dozen eggs} : 33 \text{ eggs}$$

$$12x = 33$$

$$x = 2.75 \text{ or } 3 \text{ dozen eggs}$$

EXAMPLE 2

A doctor gives a patient a prescription that instructs the patient to take 2 tablets every 4 hours. The prescription orders 120 tablets to be issued. How long will the prescription last if the tablets are taken as ordered?

$$2 \text{ tablets every } 4 \text{ hr} = 12 \text{ tablets per } 24 \text{ hr} = 12 \text{ tablets per day}$$

$$12 \text{ tablets} : 1 \text{ day} = 120 \text{ tablets} : x \text{ days}$$

$$12x = 120$$

$$x = 10 \text{ days}$$

Percentage Problems

EXAMPLE 1

Margaret bought a coat on sale. The list price of the coat was $245. She paid $200 for the coat. What was the rate of discount on the coat?

Cost of coat = $245

Discount price of coat = $200

Amount of discount = $45

$$\frac{\text{Amount of discount}}{\text{Cost}} = \frac{45}{245} = 0.1836 = 18.4\%$$

EXAMPLE 2

The Smith family budget allows 15% of monthly income for eating out and entertainment for themselves and their seven children. Mr. Smith contributes $2,400 a month to the budget, and his wife contributes $2,700 a month. How much can the Smith family spend a month on eating out and entertainment?

Mr. Smith = $2,400

Mrs. Smith = $2,700

Total monthly amount to budget = $5,100

Entertainment percentage = 15% = 0.15

(Total amount to budget)(Percentage) = ($5,100)(0.15) = $765.00

Sales Problems

EXAMPLE 1

Basketballs cost a store manager $15 each. He plans to sell the basketballs at a profit of 40% over the cost. His overhead on each basketball is $3. What is the selling price of the basketballs?

Basketball cost = $15

Overhead = $3

Profit = 40% = 0.40

Selling price = Cost + Overhead + Profit

Selling price = $15 + $3 + ($15)(0.40)

Selling price = $15 + $3 + $6

Selling price = $24.00

EXAMPLE 2

The Roundrock Pet Company had sales in the amount of $6,500 for one week. The cost of the merchandise sold was $3,800. The store's overhead was 15% of sales. How much profit was made during the week?

Amount of sales = $6,500

Cost of merchandise = $3,800

Overhead = 15% = 0.15

If Selling price = Cost + Overhead + Profit, then

Profit = Selling price − Cost − Overhead

Profit = $6,500 − $3,800 − (0.15)($6,500)

Profit = $6,500 − $3,800 − $975

Profit = $1,725

Mixture Problems

EXAMPLE 1

The adult dinner theater sold 198 tickets. Adult tickets sold for $15.25 and student tickets for $10.25. If the income for the dinner theater was $2,629.50, how many of each type ticket were sold?

Set up a table to solve this problem.

	Number of Tickets	**Cost of Tickets**	**Total Income**
Adult Tickets	x	$15.25	$15.25x
Student Tickets	$198 - x$	$10.25	$10.25(198 - x)$
Total Tickets	$15.25x$	$10.25(198 - x)$	$2,629.50

Ticket income = Adult ticket income + Student ticket income

$2,629.50 = 15.25x + 10.25(198 - x)$

$2,629.50 = 15.25x + 2,029.50 - 10.25x$

$2,629.50 = 5x + 2,029.50$

$600 = 5x$

$120 = x$ (Adult tickets sold)

$78 = 198 - x$ (Student tickets sold)

EXAMPLE 2

A jar contains four colors of candy. One fourth of the candy is red in color, one fifth of the candy is green, one fifth of the candy is yellow, and the remaining 30 pieces of candy are orange. How many pieces of candy are in the jar?

$\frac{1}{4}$ = red candies $\frac{1}{5}$ = green candies

$\frac{1}{5}$ = yellow candies   30 = orange candies

x = total pieces of candy

Total pieces of candy = #red + #green + #yellow + #orange

$$x = \left(\frac{1}{4}x\right) + \left(\frac{1}{5}x\right) + \left(\frac{1}{5}x\right) + 30$$

$20x = 5x + 4x + 4x + 600$

$20x = 13x + 600$

$7x = 600$

$x = 85.7 = 86$ pieces of candy

Tax Problems

EXAMPLE 1

Jonathan works for Zippies Burgers. His weekly salary is $380. His employer deducts 4% of his salary for Social Security, 5.25% for state withholding tax, and 7% for federal withholding tax. Jonathan uses direct deposit and an additional $50 is deducted and put into a savings account before the money is put into his checking account. How much money goes into Jonathan's checking account each week?

Total weekly salary (WS) = $380

Social Security deduction (SS) = 4% = $380(0.04) = $15.20

State deduction (SD) = 5.25% = 0.0525 = $380(0.0525) = $19.95

Federal deduction (FD) = 7% = $380(0.07) = $26.60

Savings account deduction (SAD) = $50

Checking account deposit = WS – (SS + SD + FD + SAD)

Checking account deposit = $380 – ($15.20 + $19.95 + $26.60 + $50)

Checking account deposit = $380 – $111.75

Checking account deposit = $268.25

EXAMPLE 2

Wanda buys a lamp for $67. The sales tax is 8.7754%. What is the total cost of her purchase?

Total cost = Cost of lamp + tax

Total cost = $67 + ($67)(0.087754)

Total cost = $67 + $5.8795

Total cost = $72.88

Geometry Problems

EXAMPLE 1

In $\triangle ABC$, the measure of $\angle A$ is five times the measure of $\angle B$. The measure of $\angle C$ is three times the measure of $\angle B$. What is the measure of each of the angles of the triangle?

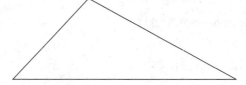

$\angle B = x$

$\angle A = 5x$

$\angle C = 3x$

$\angle B + \angle A + \angle C = 180°$

$x + 5x + 3x = 180°$

$9x = 180°$

$x = 20° = \angle B$

$5x = 100° = \angle A$

$3x = 60° = \angle C$

EXAMPLE 2

A carpenter is painting a house and needs access to the second-story windows. The bottom of the windows are 15 feet from the ground. The nearest a ladder can be safely placed to the house is 7 feet. The house is at a right angle to the ground. How long a ladder does the carpenter need to access the second-story windows?

Draw a diagram to help solve the problem.

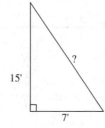

a = house = 15 feet

b = ground = 7 feet

c = ladder = unknown feet

$a^2 + b^2 = c^2$

$15^2 + 7^2 = c^2$

$225 + 49 = c^2$

$274 = c^2$

$\sqrt{274} = 16.6 = c$

16.6 feet = c = length of ladder

Insurance Problems

EXAMPLE 1

Martha is considering purchasing a life insurance policy. The annual premium rate on $10,000 worth of life insurance is $25 per $1,000. What is the annual cost of Martha's premium?

Policy worth = $10,000

Premium rate = $25/$1,000

$25 : $1,000 :: x : $10,000

$1,000x = 250,000$

$x = \$250$

EXAMPLE 2

A boat is insured against fire for 85% of its value. The boat has a value of $85,000 and the premium rate is $15 per $1,000. What is the annual premium for the boat?

Policy = 85% of value of boat = $72,250

Value of boat = $85,000

Premium rate = $15/$1,000

$15 : $1,000 :: x : $72,250

$1,000x = 1,083,750$

$x = \$1,083.75$

Investment Problems

EXAMPLE 1

Timothy owns 750 shares of Lifelong Computer stock. The stock pays an annual dividend of $22.79 per share. How much will Timothy receive in dividends this year?

number of shares = 750

dividends/share = $22.79

(750)($22.79) = $17,092.50

EXAMPLE 2

Joyce bought 110 shares of BioTech Limited at $21 a share. She sold the shares a year later at $27 a share. What is her profit after paying a commission of $40?

Original price = (110 shares)($21) = $2,310

Selling price = (110 shares)($27) = $2,970

Commission = $40

Selling price − Original price − Commission = Profit

$$\$2,970 - \$2,310 - \$40 = Profit$$

$$\$620 = Profit$$

Interest Problems

EXAMPLE 1

What is the simple interest on $15,000 invested at 10% annual rate over 3 years?

Principal = $15,000

Rate = 10% annually

Time = 3 years

Interest = Principal × Rate × Time

Interest = ($15,000)(0.10)(3)

Interest = $4,500

EXAMPLE 2

What is the simple interest on $1,800 at a 5.5% semiannual rate over 6 years?

Principal = $1800

Rate = 5.5% semiannually = 11% annually

Time = 6 years

Interest = Principal × Rate × Time

Interest = $1,800 × 0.11 × 6

Interest = $1,188

Average Problems

EXAMPLE 1

EXAMPLE 1

Mike has the following points on pop quizzes: 10, 15, 21, 7, 27, 32, 50, 50, and 50. Each quiz is worth 50 points. If 70% is a passing grade, does Mike have a passing average on quizzes?

$$\left(\frac{10+15+21+7+27+32+50+50+50}{9} \right) = 29.11 \text{ points}$$

70% of 50 = 35 points

Mike does not have a passing average on pop quizzes.

EXAMPLE 2

Tickets for the All School Play sell for $1.50, $2.50, $5.00, and $10.00. What is the average price of a ticket?

$$\frac{\$1.50+\$2.50+\$5.00+\$10.00}{4} = \$4.75$$

Dosage Problems

EXAMPLE 1

A patient is receiving cough medicine (liquid), 500 milligrams (mg) by mouth every 6 hours. The medication label reads: 250 milligrams/5 milliliters (mL). How many mL will the nurse administer for one dose?

Formula:

$$\frac{\text{Desired} \times \text{Volume}}{\text{Available}} = \text{mL per dose}$$

$$\frac{500 \text{ mg} \times 5 \text{ mL}}{250 \text{ mg}} = 10 \text{ mL}$$

The action falls under application. The nurse giving the necessary medication to assist with coughing helps the patient physiologically.

EXAMPLE 2

A dentist has his nurse administer a one time antibiotic dose to a patient with a tooth infection. The dose is 7.5 milligrams (mg) intramuscularly (IM). The medication concentration mix is 10 milligrams/milliliters (mL). How many milliliters will the nurse give to the patient for the one time dose?

Formula:

$$\frac{\text{Desired} \times \text{Volume}}{\text{Available}} = \text{mL per dose}$$

$$\frac{7.5 \text{ mg} \times 1 \text{ mL}}{10 \text{ mg}} = 0.75 \text{ mL}$$

The action falls under application. The nurse giving the necessary medication to assist with coughing helps the patient physiologically.

EXAMPLE 3

Before calculating a drug dosage for a newborn, infant, or child, the nurse should check to see if the drug has been ordered in a safe range. The physician orders gentamycin (antibiotic) 20 milligrams (mg) intramuscularly (IM) for a child 18 months old weighing 22 pounds (lb). Check a Pediatric Drug Handbook for safe dosage range.

   The Pediatric Drug Handbook states: *Maximum daily dosage of gentamycin for a child is 6–7.5 mg/kg/24 hours and divided every 8 hr.*

First: Convert pounds to kilograms (kg):

   2.2 lb = 1 kg

   $\dfrac{2.2\ lb}{1\ kg} = \dfrac{22\ lb}{x\ kg}$ $x = 10$ kg (22 lb = 10 kg)

Second: Calculate the safe dosage range for 24 hours:

   $10 \times 7.5 = 75$ mg per 24 hours

Third: Calculate the safe dosage range for each dose every 8 hours:

   $\dfrac{75\ mg}{3} = 25$ mg

The physician's dosage is within a safe range at 20 mg every 8 hours.

EXAMPLE 4

A physician orders D5%NS 1,000 milliliters (mL) to infuse over 8 hours. The nurse plans to run the infusion by intravenous (IV) pump. What rate will the nurse set the IV pump to infuse at?

Formula:

   $\dfrac{Total\ volume}{Hours} = \dfrac{1,000\ mL}{8} = 125$ mL/hour

Answer Sheet
SAMPLE TEST

Verbal Problems

1 Ⓐ Ⓑ Ⓒ Ⓓ   8 Ⓐ Ⓑ Ⓒ Ⓓ   15 Ⓐ Ⓑ Ⓒ Ⓓ
2 Ⓐ Ⓑ Ⓒ Ⓓ   9 Ⓐ Ⓑ Ⓒ Ⓓ   16 Ⓐ Ⓑ Ⓒ Ⓓ
3 Ⓐ Ⓑ Ⓒ Ⓓ   10 Ⓐ Ⓑ Ⓒ Ⓓ   17 Ⓐ Ⓑ Ⓒ Ⓓ
4 Ⓐ Ⓑ Ⓒ Ⓓ   11 Ⓐ Ⓑ Ⓒ Ⓓ   18 Ⓐ Ⓑ Ⓒ Ⓓ
5 Ⓐ Ⓑ Ⓒ Ⓓ   12 Ⓐ Ⓑ Ⓒ Ⓓ   19 Ⓐ Ⓑ Ⓒ Ⓓ
6 Ⓐ Ⓑ Ⓒ Ⓓ   13 Ⓐ Ⓑ Ⓒ Ⓓ
7 Ⓐ Ⓑ Ⓒ Ⓓ   14 Ⓐ Ⓑ Ⓒ Ⓓ

Verbal Problem Sample Test

Verbal Problem Sample Test

Directions: For each question, select the letter (A, B, C, or D) that best corresponds to your answer. Record your answers on the answer sheet on page 187.

1. A cooking class is baking cookies for a school party. Recipes A and C each yield 4 dozen cookies and require two eggs per recipe. Recipe B yields 2 dozen cookies and requires one egg per recipe. One-fifth of the total dozens of cookies will be Recipe A; two-fifths of the total dozens will be Recipe B; and 20 dozen cookies will be Recipe C. What is the total number of eggs needed to make cookies for the school party?

   CHALLENGE

   (A) 5 eggs
   (B) 12 eggs
   (C) 16 eggs
   (D) 22 eggs

2. Sarah and Rachael are sisters. Rachael is younger than Sarah by 3 years. Sarah is 5 years older than her brother, Tom, who was born in 1996. In what years were Rachael and Sarah born?

   (A) Sarah was born in 2001; Rachael was born in 1998.
   (B) Sarah was born in 2005; Rachael was born in 2003.
   (C) Sarah was born in 1999; Rachael was born in 1996.
   (D) Sarah was born in 1991; Rachael was born in 1994.

3. Directions on your bottle of cough syrup read: Take 15 ml every six hours as needed for cough. How many teaspoons (tsp) of cough medicine will you take for your cough?

   (A) 3 tsp
   (B) 9 tsp
   (C) 12 tsp
   (D) 15 tsp

4. A discount store has a video game for $76.95. A retail store has the same game for $99.00 with a 20% markdown at checkout. Which store is offering the best buy?

   (A) Retail store has better price savings by $19.80.
   (B) Discount store has better price savings by $2.25.
   (C) Retail store has better price by $6.95.
   (D) With retail store discount, the price is the same at both stores.

5. A map has a scale of 1 inch = 75 miles. Donnerville and Wright's Point are $5\frac{3}{4}$ inches apart. What is the distance, in miles, between the two locations?

   (A) 370.40 miles
   (B) 355.35 miles
   (C) 450.07 miles
   (D) 431.25 miles

6. Glynnis has $45.00 for the purchase of a lamp. She finds a lamp with a price tag of $69.99 marked 25% off today only. Sales tax is 6.788%. Does Glynnis have enough money to make the purchase?

   (A) No, Glynnis needs $3.05 to purchase the lamp.
   (B) Yes, Glynnis will have one cent remaining after the lamp purchase.
   (C) No, Glynnis needs $11.05 to purchase the lamp.
   (D) Yes, Glynnis will have $13.94 remaining after the lamp purchase.

7. Tuition at a community college increased from $55.00 to $62.00 per semester hour. What is the percentage of increase?

(A) 1.13%
(B) 7.0%
(C) 8.87%
(D) 12.73%

8. A nurse is gauze to dress 3 wounds. He has a length of gauze 5 feet long that needs to be cut into three pieces with two of the three pieces 2 inches longer than the remaining piece. Determine the lengths of the three pieces.

CHALLENGE

(A) 1 length = 10 inches;
    2 lengths = 25 inches each
(B) 1 length = 18.7 inches;
    2 lengths = 20.7 inches each
(C) 1 length = 20.0 inches;
    2 lengths = 22.0 inches each
(D) 1 length = 26 inches;
    2 lengths = 28 inches each

9. A large photograph measuring 12 inches in length and 8 inches in width needs to be reduced so the length will be 8 inches. Determine the width of the photograph when reduced.

(A) $5\frac{1}{3}$ inches
(B) 4 inches
(C) $3\frac{1}{3}$ inches
(D) 2 inches

10. Two runners start running toward each other from different points in the county at the same time. The two points are 34 miles apart. Runner A averages 3 miles per hour and reaches the meeting point in 5 hours. Runner B misses a turn and runs 10 extra miles. What distance did each runner cover?

(A) Runner A runs 15 miles; Runner B runs 19 miles.
(B) Runner A runs 15 miles; Runner B runs 29 miles.
(C) Runner A runs 11.3 miles; runner B runs 22.7 miles.
(D) Runner A runs 11.3 miles; Runner B runs 32.7 miles.

11. The ratio of concentrated liquid hair color to the mixing agent is 2:5. If 3 ounces of hair color are in the package, how many ounces of the mixing agent are needed to prepare the hair coloring solution?

(A) 4 ounces
(B) 7.5 ounces
(C) 10 ounces
(D) 15.6 ounces

12. A student wants to know what grade he needs to make on the final exam to have a grade of 80% in a course. His grade on the first exam was 65%, second exam was 85%, and third exam was 77%. The first three exams are each worth 20% of the overall grade with the final exam worth 40%. What grade does the student need to make on the final exam to have a grade of 80% in the course?

(A) 54.6%
(B) 75.6%
(C) 80.0%
(D) 86.5%

13. A farmer needs to buy chicken wire for a coop he is building for his pigeons. The front, floor, and roof of the coop will be wood with the remaining three sides (2 long sides and 1 short side) in chicken wire. The length of the coop is 15 feet, with the width and height each 10 feet. Rolls of chicken wire are 5 feet in height and 100 feet in length. What length of chicken wire does the farmer need to purchase for his pigeon coop? *Draw a diagram to help solve the problem.*

(A) 20 feet
(B) 40 feet
(C) 80 feet
(D) 100 feet

CHALLENGE

14. An ancient statue is insured for 90% of its value. The statue has a value of $100,000. The annual premium rate is $20.00 per $1,000 of value. What is the annual premium for the statue?

    (A) $18,000
    (B) $9,000
    (C) $4,500
    (D) $1,500

15. Martin is planning to paint four rooms at the homeless shelter. Rooms 110 and 113 are 14 feet in length, 12 feet in width, and 9 feet in height. Rooms 212 and 216 are 25 feet in length, 22 feet wide, and 10 feet in height. Determine the number of square feet to be covered.

    (A) 1232.1 square feet
    (B) 2277 square feet
    (C) 2816 square feet
    (D) 3000.5 square feet

    CHALLENGE

16. The physician ordered Demerol 45 milligrams (mg) intramuscularly (IM) every 6 hours (hr) for pain. The medication label reads 75 mg/mL. How many milliliters (mL) will the nurse administer to the patient?

    (A) 2 mL
    (B) 1 mL
    (C) 0.7 mL
    (D) 0.6 mL

17. The medication label reads Zantac 150 milligrams (mg) per tablet. The patient's order is written for 0.3 grams (gm) by mouth (PO) daily. How many tablets will the nurse administer to the patient?

    (A) ½ tablet
    (B) 1.5 tablets
    (C) 2 tablets
    (D) 2.5 tablets

18. A patient is to receive Heparin 15,000 units. The medication is available as 25,000 units/mL. How many milliliters (mL) of Heparin will the patient receive?

    (A) 0.45 mL
    (B) 0.5 mL
    (C) 0.56 mL
    (D) 0.6 mL

19. The nurse is starting an intravenous (IV) on a patient who is to receive sodium chloride 1,000 milliliters (mL) of solution to infuse over 12 hours by IV pump. The IV will infuse at how many mL per hour?

    (A) 83 mL/hr
    (B) 82 mL/hr
    (C) 80 mL/hr
    (D) 79 mL/hr

Verbal Problem Sample Test Answer Key

1. **(D)** x = Total dozens of cookies

   Recipe A = $\frac{1}{5}$ or 20% of the total dozens of cookies (makes 4 dozen; uses 2 eggs)

   Recipe B = $\frac{2}{5}$ or 40% of the total dozens of cookies (makes 2 dozen; uses 1 egg)

   Recipe C = 20 dozen cookies (makes 4 dozen; uses 2 eggs)

   $x = 20\%(x) + 40\%(x) + 20$ dozen cookies
   $x = .20x + .40x + 20$
   $.40x = 20$
   $x = 50$ dozen cookies

   Recipe A = 20% of 50 dozen = 10 dozen = 2 recipes $\times$ 2 eggs = 4 eggs
   Recipe B = 40% of 50 dozen = 20 dozen = 10 recipes $\times$ 1 egg = 10 eggs
   Recipe C = 20 dozen = 4 recipes $\times$ 2 eggs = 8 eggs

   4 eggs + 10 eggs + 8 eggs = 22 eggs

2. **(D)** 1996 = year Tom was born
   1996 – 5 = 1991, or year Sarah was born
   1991 + 3 = 1994, or year Rachael was born

3. **(A)** 1 tsp = 5 ml
   x = teaspoons of cough syrup to administer

   1 tsp : 5 ml = x tsp : 15 ml
   x = 3 tsp

4. **(B)** Discount store price = $76.95
   Retail store price = $99.00 with 20% discount at checkout

   $99.00 \times 20\% = 99 \times .20 = $19.80
   $99.00 - $19.80 = $79.20

   $79.20 - $76.95 = $2.25

5. **(D)** 1 inch = 75 miles
   x = distance in miles between locations
   $5\frac{3}{4}$ inches = measured distance from Donnerville and Wright's Point

   1 inch : 75 miles = 5.75 inches : x miles
   x = 431.25 miles

6. **(C)** *Amount* of money Glynnis has to spend = $45.00
Price of lamp = $69.99
Sale price of lamp = $52.49
Sale mark down = 25% or ($17.50)
Sales tax = 6.788% or ($3.45)

Total cost = $\left[\text{Sale price of lamp}\right]$ + Sales tax
Total cost of lamp = $56.05

Cost of lamp – Amount Glynnis has to spend = $56.05 − $45.00 = $ 11.05
Glynnis does not have enough money for the purchase.

7. **(D)** Original tuition = $55.00 per semester hour
New tuition = $62.00 per semester hour

New tuition – Original tuition = $62.00 − $55.00 = $7.00 increase in tuition

$\dfrac{\text{Increase in tuition}}{\text{Original tuition}} = \dfrac{7}{55} =$ 12.727 = 12.73% increase in tuition

8. **(B)** Length of gauze = 5 feet or 60 inches
Length of one shorter piece in inches = x inches
Lengths of two longer pieces in feet or inches = $2(x + 2$ inches$)$

$$x + 2\left(x + 2 \text{ inches}\right) = 60 \text{ inches}$$
$$x + 2x + 4 = 60$$
$$3x + 4 = 60$$
$$3x = 56$$
$$x = 18.65 = 18.7$$
$$x + 2 = 20.7$$

9. **(A)** *Original* photo = 12 inches by 8 inches
Reduced photo length = 8 inches
Reduced photo width = x

Original length : Original width = Reduced length : Reduced width
$$12 : 8 = 8 : x$$
$$12x = 64$$
$$x = 5.33 \text{ inches}$$

10. **(B)** Distance between 2 points = 34 miles
Runner A average rate = 3 mph
Runner A time = 5 hr
Runner A distance = D_A
Runner B distance = D_B

Runner A: $D_A = R \cdot T$ Runner B: $D_B = 34 − D_A + 10$
$D_A = 3 \cdot 5$ $D_B = 29$ miles
$D_A = 15$ miles

11. **(B)** *Hair* color = 2 parts
Mixing agent = 5 parts
Hair color in package = 3 ounces
Ounces of mixing agent needed = x

$$2 \text{ parts} : 3 \text{ ounces} = 5 \text{ parts} : x \text{ ounces}$$
$$x = 7.5 \text{ ounces}$$

12. **(D)** Exam 1 = 65%
Exam 2 = 85%
Exam 3 = 77%
Weight of each exam = 20%
Weight of final exam = 40%
Final exam grade = x

$$\left(\textit{Exam } 1 \cdot 20\%\right) + \left(\text{Exam } 2 \cdot 20\%\right) + \left(\text{Exam } 3 \cdot 20\%\right) + \left(x \cdot 40\%\right) = 80\%$$
$$x = 86.5\%$$

13. **(C)** *Length of each* long *side* = 15 feet
Width of one short side = 10 feet
Height = 10 feet
Roll of chicken wire = 100 feet by 5 feet
$x = (P \cdot 2)$ = Length of chicken wire

Perimeter = 2(length) + width
P = 2(15) + 10
P = 40 feet

$x = P \cdot 2 = 40 \cdot 2 = 80$ feet

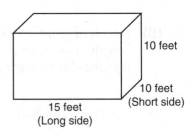

10 feet

10 feet
(Short side)

15 feet
(Long side)

14. **(A)** Value of statue = $100,000
Insured value = 90%
Annual premium rate = $20.00/$1,000
x = annual premium

$100,000 • 90% = $90,000.00

$20 : $1,000 = x : $90,000
$18,000 = x

15. **(C)**   Rooms 110 & 113: Length = 14 feet; Width = 12 feet; Height = 9 feet
     Rooms 212 & 216: Length = 25 feet; Width = 22 feet; Height = 10 feet

$$\text{Area}_1 = \left[2\left(\text{Width} \bullet \text{Height}\right) + 2\left(\text{Length} \bullet \text{Height}\right) \right] \bullet 2 \text{ rooms}$$
$$A_1 = \left[2\left(12 \bullet 9\right) + 2\left(14 \bullet 9\right) \right] \bullet 2$$
$$A_1 = 468 \text{ square feet} \bullet 2 = 936 \text{ square feet}$$

$$\text{Area}_2 = \left[2\left(\text{Width} \bullet \text{Height}\right) + 2\left(\text{Length} \bullet \text{Height}\right) \right] \bullet 2 \text{ rooms}$$
$$A_2 = 2\left(22 \bullet 10\right) + 2\left(25 \bullet 10\right)$$
$$A_2 = 940 \text{ square feet} \bullet 2 \text{ rooms} = 1880 \text{ square feet}$$

$$A_1 + A_2 = 936 + 1880 = 2816 \text{ square feet}$$

16. **(D)** $\dfrac{\text{Desired} \times \text{Volume}}{\text{Available}} = \text{mL per dose}$

$$\frac{45 \text{ mg} \times 1 \text{ mL}}{75 \text{ mg}} = 0.6 \text{ mL}$$

17. **(C)**   Convert 0.3 gm to mg

mg means "milligram"; 0.3 gm = 300 mg

$$\frac{\text{Desired} \times \text{Volume}}{\text{Available}} = \text{mL per dose}$$

$$\frac{300 \text{ mg} \times 1 \text{ tab}}{150 \text{ mg}} = 2 \text{ tablets}$$

18. **(D)** $\dfrac{\text{Desired} \times \text{Volume}}{\text{Available}} = \text{mL per dose}$

$$\frac{15,000 \text{ units} \times 1 \text{ mL}}{25,000 \text{ units}} = 0.6 \text{ mL}$$

19. **(A)**   Sodium chloride IV solution 1,000 mL to infuse over 12 hours. The IV will infuse by IV pump. The rate will be set by the nurse.

$$\frac{1,000 \text{ mL}}{12 \text{ hr}} = 83.3 \text{ mL}$$

Science Review

The study of science is divided into two basic areas of thought: the physical sciences and the organic sciences. The physical sciences are concerned with the properties of events, such as the weather or the behavior of rocks or of elements of matter. The study of the physical sciences can be thought of as the study of nonliving things. For example, physics deals with the behavior of energy and matter, waves and particles, motion, and forces such as electromagnetism and thermodynamics. Scientists are concerned with physics when they study things ranging from the behavior of small particles of matter to principles of energy exchange in the larger universe. Scientists are concerned with physics as they seek to understand the underlying principles that make the universe work. By contrast, the organic sciences are concerned with living things (those things that perform certain sets of behaviors). These living things might be plants or animals or some of the smallest known living things, the viruses.

The study of either type of science can become lengthy and complex. What you will review in connection with this chapter is substantial and will give you background information in science, not only for the purpose of handling nursing entrance testing but also for a lifetime in a profession based very solidly on a broad-based understanding of almost all the sciences. Nursing is a profession that borrows from many other sources. Consequently, everything that you have learned about the sciences to this point will be useful. It will provide a foundation for nursing proficiency throughout the years ahead.

This chapter builds on the simpler and smaller and moves on to the more complex and more organized. It begins with a review of the world of nonliving things, with an emphasis on their physical properties. The chapter then proceeds to the study of living things, beginning with classification. Using the concepts behind organic chemistry, we will look at the behavior of the smallest particles and cells within living bodies. Then we will transfer our attention to the natural clustering of associated cells into tissues, organs, systems, and the entire organism. This chapter reviews both structure and function within organisms. Finally, we will consider some useful principles from systems theory, sociology, and psychology, which will allow you to place the study of humans and other living things into an even broader perspective. Test items occur throughout the text material.

In addition to the material provided in this chapter, the interested reader might want to consider searching the Internet for a simple anatomy and physiology review book. There are a number on the market that will help to form a baseline of knowledge for later physiology-based classes once you are in nursing school as well as to serve as a basic review when you later take the licensure test once your coursework in nursing school is complete. Books that begin with titles such as "Key Facts" or "Fundamentals" are usually tailored for review purposes.

As you are studying for your nursing entrance examination, bear in mind that some of these tests can be quite simple. Some tests require only the ability to read science paragraphs for comprehension. In essence, the test taker needs no prior knowledge of science. Nevertheless, even when taking this type of nursing entrance examination, practice with the problems presented here offers you an extra measure of confidence.

Nonliving Things

The study of nonliving things begins with the study of physics. Physics studies the physical principles of our perceived reality—the world, the universe, whatever we can conjecture might exist. We study physics to attempt to understand the behavior of matter and energy and the relationship of time to existence. In the study of physics, we attempt to explain the small and invisible forces and objects in our world as well as the enormous forces within an extremely large and complex universe. It may relate to the present as we examine the current generated within electrical connections, or it may involve principles related to the origin of the universe, an event of long ago. As we begin to deal with some of the physical principles most pertinent to nursing's view of reality, let's look at what constitutes life and nonlife.

Entropy and Negentropy

One of the most basic questions that has surfaced during humanity's study of the world around it is the question of life versus nonlife. What makes the difference between living and nonliving entities and how did life start? Without considering the answers provided by the world's major religions and its great philosophers, it is clear that there is no simple answer.

One explanation involves entropy and negentropy. Entropy is the tendency of matter to return to a state of stasis, or nonlife. Because entropy is frequently thought of in terms of randomness, it can also be defined as the amount of disorder that exists within something. For example, a rock is not alive. It does not take in matter, put out any sort of byproduct, have any feedback mechanisms, move under its own power, or reproduce. This rock, which is in a relative state of entropy, has no sense of sentience or purposefulness, nor does it have an orderly organization of systems of matter or energy within it. However, even matter in this state has a property known as energy. Even though a rock as a whole doesn't move about under its own power, its individual components, the atoms, have moving parts. However, for the rock to move away from this relative state of entropy, there must be an infusion of energy. More orderly and organized systems and subsystems require more energy. The rock is also a solid; it possesses a distinct form. A rock looks like a rock. The form of a solid object assists with recognition. Objects in a relative state of entropy also have gravity.

The opposite of entropy is negentropy. As things move farther from entropy, they engage in processes that require an increasing amount of matter and energy exchange and internal manipulation. We do not know what occurred on our particular planet that stimulated the earth's ancient cosmic soup to form the first earth-bound, living entities. But it is something for the person acting as caregiver to consider. Even though human beings use the term *energy* in different ways, they seem to feel that they possess greater or lesser amounts of physical energy at different times. This feeling of having either great energy or low energy is probably an intricate feedback mechanism put in place to alert people to the need to restore their energy. Although this use of the term is different from what pure scientists mean by energy, perhaps the two conventions are related. As a nurse, you will find yourself in situations in which your ability to preserve or enhance the patient's relative energy levels will make a positive difference.

To return to the question of what distinguishes entropy from negentropy, and the living from the nonliving, scientists have tried to duplicate what are thought to be the ancient conditions from which life arose on earth. But, despite repeated trials using electrical or other forms of energy, they have had no success. It would seem that this ancient mystery will remain just that. It is known, however, that entropy tends to increase or to stay constant and that there is a natural tendency for things to return to a state of disorder. Knowing this, we can consider some of the other elemental properties of matter and energy of interest to those in the health sciences.

Physical Forces: Gravity, Friction, Motion, and Energy

All matter possesses gravity, the property of attraction. Larger objects have more gravity than do smaller objects. Entities that are larger attract more strongly. That is why humans remain on the surface of the earth, rather than floating away into space. The force of the earth's gravity keeps us locked to the planet's surface. The oceans remain in place because of gravity. The apple falls from the tree because of gravity. The moon circles the earth because the earth is larger and attracts the moon to it, in a looser sort of sense.

Gravity is also involved in nurses' daily dealings with patients. As human beings, we understand gravity instinctively. From an early age, we know that we cannot fly through the air and that an object will land on the floor if we drop it. As we become older, we realize that we can be injured if we fall or if we cause our bones or joints to act in ways that defy gravity too intensely or at too much of an angle from a straight line. This understanding encompasses an entire branch of physics that deals with vectors, or angles of motion or force. The nurse learns early that there are angles at which to apply force that will minimize the risk of injury.

As nurses, we learn that, when assisting others who cannot move independently, we risk injury from the extra weight to be moved. Humans are the only living creatures who spend most of a lifetime walking erect. This places stress upon areas of our bodies, particularly the muscles and connective tissues of the back. Nurses spend much of their time around patients' bedsides lifting, bending, stretching, reaching, pushing, and pulling. This can strain already-stressed back muscles.

An entire field of study, involving the principles of gravity, has evolved to help the caregiver avoid injury from dealing with heavy weights and acts involving repetitive motion. Physical therapists and nurses learn the principles of body mechanics early in their careers.

The following rules illustrate the practical application of these principles:

1. When dealing with weights, pulling, pushing, and pivoting are more desirable than lifting.
2. If lifting, bend from the knees and use a broad base of support by placing your feet apart. Hold the object to be lifted close to the body.
3. If in doubt about being able to accomplish the task without injury to self or another, get a second person to assist.
4. Use right angles. If pulling an object toward you, bend from the knees in order to keep your back straight and pull directly to you, rather than at an angle.
5. Any repetitive motion may be associated with eventual injury.

Levers, metal weights, and pulleys may also provide assistance to those caring for patients. For example, one of the machines used to lift a patient from the bed to a chair is a lift. It uses a lever system to hoist a patient into the air. The lift can then be maneuvered over a chair or the chair can come to the patient. Using this machine prevents caregivers from intensively using their own back muscles in repetitively lifting or pivoting with patients.

An understanding of the use of such things as weights and pulleys in maintaining a straight line of pull is important. When a patient fractures a leg or arm bone it is necessary to remain in bed to avoid placing pressure on the fracture and to align the fractured ends in a manner that involves a straight line and approximation of the bone ends. In the case of a leg bone, this is achieved by attaching a metal weight to a rope device and hanging the weight over the end of the bed. When the rope device is attached to the fractured bone end that is farther from the center of the body, the weight exerts a straight line pull. This force relieves pain and overcomes the tendency of the body's muscles and ligaments to exert pull in various other directions while healing occurs. This set of devices, known as traction, can be released when the fracture has healed. In some cases, however, traction is unnecessary or undesirable, and alternate methods to stabilize the bone ends are used. Traction devices use the force of gravity to stabilize a fracture. In the case of alternate devices, such as casts or internal placement of metal rods, plates, or screws, stability is achieved despite gravity.

The principles of friction and kinetic energy are also useful for nurses. For example, friction involves the propensity of relatively rougher objects rubbing against each other to slow or stop, or to require greater energy to maintain in motion, as compared to smoother objects' propensity to keep going. For example, if you rolled a play car across a smooth surface, such as a tiled kitchen floor, it would go farther than if you rolled it across the same kitchen floor to which a layer of sand has been added. The smooth floor offers less friction and so the object in motion remains in motion longer when the same amount of force is applied. Friction is also what causes your car to come to a stop when you take your foot off the gas pedal. Friction generates heat, such as when one rubs one's hands briskly together.

Let us consider another example. The space between the lining over the lungs and the inner lining of the chest cavity is normally smooth. The surfaces glide smoothly over each other as we breathe. The breathing process is relatively effortless. When these lining surfaces become roughened from inflammation, a grating, painful, effort-filled breathing pattern results. More energy is required to perform the act of breathing. Internally, body cavities and internal tube systems are lined with smooth substances. In their healthy state, heart valves, the interior of blood vessels, the surfaces of our bones' joints, and the small air sacs of the lungs are all smooth and even have slight coatings of liquid lubricants, when necessary. When these surfaces become roughened, they do not operate as well and may become permanently damaged.

On a larger scale, nurses working around patients pay attention to friction when moving the relatively helpless older patients toward the head of the bed. If there is too much friction between the patients' skin and the bed linens, the fragile skin surfaces may be injured. Therefore, a slight lift, preferably with another person to assist, is the wiser course of action.

What does classical mechanics have to do with nursing? Nurses are guided by principles of motion, force, and energy. For the nurse moving the patient in bed, inertia and force have a practical application. When a nurse starts to move a patient in bed, placing the patient in slight motion by rocking gently in the direction of the pull prior to the larger effort of the actual move will make the move much easier for patient and nurse. This preparation is similar to that of the bobsledder, or skier, who rocks back and forth at the starting gate to build momentum prior to shoving off down the hill. In both cases, there is an effort to overcome inertia, or the tendency for an object at rest to stay that way.

In all of these cases, the nurse's energy is used to assist another in performing acts that could not be performed unaided. It is important for the nurse to conserve her own energies and to find the best ways to exert force.

Physical Properties of Liquids and Gases: Pressure Principles

Gravity also causes liquids to run downhill. Consider liquids that flow through tube systems. When the liquid is high in the air, it will move rapidly to seek the lowest possible level. When dealing with intravenous solutions infusing into patients' veins via gravity, the nurse can influence the rate of flow by elevating or lowering the height of the solution. The higher the solution, the faster it will flow.

Pressure principles are also important to nurses who deal with liquids or with gas exchange. Our respiratory system could not function without changing pressures. Additionally, many of the devices used in modern health care employ pressure principles to move liquids and gases from one place to another. For example, in order for air to enter our lungs, the diaphragm, a band of tissue that resembles a round trampoline, drops downward slightly and the musculature between our ribs helps to expand the space in which our lungs rest. This expansion creates a negative pressure that causes air to enter from the higher pressure atmosphere of the world outside. Air rushes in, and we have the sensation of inhaling. If we consciously want to inhale more deeply, we can even concentrate on expanding the space more fully and for a longer time.

Consequently, when dealing with pressure, we can see that fluids and gases tend to flow from an area of relatively greater pressure to an area of relatively lesser pressure. This principle also applies to suction devices such as those used during surgery or in the emergency room. Typically, a wall device creates negative pressure when turned on. Anyone using a length of tubing attached to the negative pressure area of the wall will find that air, liquids, and even small solid objects will be sucked through the tube and into the area of less pressure. For example, on televised hospital shows, the doctor often calls for suction and places something that resembles an inflated plastic straw near an area from which liquid must be sucked up. If you placed your hand or fingertips over such a tube, your skin and the underlying tissues would adhere slightly to the tube. Fortunately, however, even when the wall suction is turned to the strongest setting, the adherence is not as strong as it would be if you were to touch a frozen metal ice tray with your fingertips.

Tubes attached to suction devices are used in a wide variety of medical equipment. For example, if the chest cavity cannot maintain enough negative pressure for air to enter and leave the little air sacs of the lung, the lung will not work effectively. To drain away any air or liquid that might have accumulated, chest tubes connected to an elaborate, relatively fail-safe suction device and drainage system (nor directly attached to suction) are used. The tubes are removed only after a condition of negative pressure is reestablished within the space between lungs and inner rib cage. The nurse working with such a system must be aware that, should the patient with chest tubes suffer respiratory distress, the negative pressure in the patient's chest may have been interrupted. Perhaps the tubing has become kinked or something has happened to the wall suction or drainage device. An understanding of negative pressure principles will help fix the problem.

Waves, Particles, and Fields

A final important set of physical principles involves wave and particle motion—part of the larger study of quantum mechanics. Understanding these principles will help you explain the unexplainable, in some cases, and appreciate such things as speech, hearing, and sight.

Sound and light both move in waves. Our eyes and ears are attuned to taking in such waves, feeding them to specialized receptors located in relatively protected areas of the body, and translating them into signals that will be delivered to and interpreted by the brain. Our eyes and ears are specialized receptor mechanisms attuned to picking up certain types of waves. Sensitive receptor cells at the back of our eyes pick up light waves. Sensitive receptor cells in our inner ears pick up sound waves. These two types of waves differ enough that our specialized receptor cells do not confuse them.

In addition to being bombarded by waves, objects are said to be surrounded by fields. An electromagnetic field, for example, lies above and surrounds the earth's surface. This field causes radio waves to remain close enough to the earth to be picked up by specialized receivers. Were it not for the earth's electromagnetic field, mass communication might be exceedingly difficult.

Within the body, our nervous system transmits impulses of positively or negatively charged particles along specialized conductor pathways. Even our hearts rely on the movement of these transmissions to beat in a rhythmic and coordinated way.

In order to function, humans are dependent on fields, waves, and the movement of charged particles. We know quite a bit about how they operate in our bodies, but there are some fields that scientists seem to know very little about. For example, earlier in this century, the Soviet Union's scientists used specialized photographic techniques called Kirilian photography to document the presence of energy fields around human beings, plants, and other living objects. These fields appeared in altered form depending on the relative health of the entity they surrounded. This was the origin of the idea that plants enjoy being spoken to.

We could easily dismiss these specialized fields as a photographic anomaly, except that certain human physical evidence makes it difficult to disregard. Consider the individual who has had a limb amputated but still feels the presence of the limb for weeks afterward. The limb itches or burns or otherwise seems to be sending neurologic signals, and when photographed using Kirilian photographic techniques, the field that used to take the shape of the limb persists in a form that would indicate the limb was still there. Therefore, the nurse caring for such a patient will need to pay attention to such physical feelings.

Finally, those working around equipment used in health care institutions need a working knowledge of electromagnetic fields. Electric current will seek ground level. If a more convenient pathway is not available, it may pass through a human being connected to an electrical supply. In those cases when low amounts of current are involved, this is not a large problem, but in other cases it may be. This is why patients must not use home electrical equipment in their hospital rooms unless it has been approved or is grounded through a specialized wall circuit.

In modern operating rooms, electrostatic charges can be dangerous. Some of the gases used to anesthetize patients or to supplement patient oxygen supplies can be explosive under the right conditions. Therefore, personnel wear shoe covers and are able to assess the relative amount of charge through a specialized metering system.

A working, practical knowledge of these few physical principles will help you as a nurse to maintain safety in patient care areas. Safety involves protecting both the patient and yourself. Teaching a family member safe ways in which to reposition a bedridden person will be necessary for those who must care for that person at home. The family of a restless teenager in traction may need to bring in home audio and video equipment. As the caregiver, you can facilitate the safe use of this equipment by arranging for timely inspection by hospital maintenance personnel.

Practice with Science Questions

Directions: Review the material on physical science and then answer the following questions.

1. Which phrase describes negentropy?

   (A) A state of relative disorder.
   (B) A state of increasing randomness.
   (C) A condition of order and purposefulness.
   (D) The typical state of a rock.

2. After an earthquake, you and another caregiver must act quickly to remove an unconscious patient from a bed and then away from a collapsing area of the room. Using principles of gravity and body mechanics, select the course of action from the following list that will result in the greatest chance of safety for all three persons involved.

(A) Leave the patient alone. Perhaps that side of the hospital will not collapse any farther.
(B) With you at the head and the other caregiver at the feet of the patient, lift the person and carry from the room.
(C) With caregivers at one side of the bed, slide the patient to the floor and drag from the room.
(D) With you at the head and the other caregiver at the foot, lift the patient using the underlying sheet pulled tautly and close to your bodies, and, using the sheet as an assist device, remove the patient from the area.

3. Knowing that liquids flow in a downward direction, where should you place the collecting receptacle for a tubing device that is draining fluid from a body cavity?

(A) Below the level of the body.
(B) At the level of the body.
(C) Above the level of the body.
(D) It does not matter.

4. You are working with a glass bottle (a vial) containing liquid medication. You will need to insert a syringe with a needle attached through the rubber diaphragm at the top of the bottle. As you draw back the inner syringe barrel, medicine will leave the bottle, since liquid flows into the negative pressure space created in the syringe. Which of the following measures will make it easier to suck liquid into the syringe?

(A) Shake the medicine vial vigorously before beginning.
(B) Refrigerate the liquid medicine.
(C) Insert air into the bottle before you draw back the syringe's inner barrel.
(D) Withdraw any excess air from the bottle before you draw back on the syringe.

5. Which of the following areas of study might explain why acupuncture seems to be effective in some cases?

(A) Gravity and attraction.
(B) The sciences of waves, fields, and electromagnetic forces.
(C) Psychology and sociology.
(D) Kinesthesiology and body mechanics.

6. Your neighbor hurt her hand while gardening and it is bleeding heavily. Using your knowledge of physics principles, which is the best initial action?

    (A) Tell her not to move. Run to the telephone to call emergency medical services.
    (B) Rinse the area with the nearby garden hose. The cold water should stop the bleeding.
    (C) Wrap the clean kerchief from your pocket around the forearm above the wound and tie it very tightly.
    (D) Grab the clean kerchief from your pocket and apply direct pressure over the wound. Raise the arm higher than your neighbor's heart.

Answers:

1. **(C)** Entropy is randomness and disorder. Negentropy is order.

2. **(D)** This technique protects the two rescuers from back injury or strain, while rescuing the patient from an untenable situation.

3. **(A)** Bedside drainage, with the collection container lower than the body, fosters gravity-assisted flow while preventing backflow.

4. **(C)** Inserting air into the bottle increases pressure inside the bottle and eases extraction of the liquid.

5. **(B)** Acupuncture is based on principles of energy flow and, in some cases, relies on weak currents generated by electricity or local friction.

6. **(D)** Direct pressure is safest and is usually the technique to try first. Raising the arm allows gravity to slightly slow the flow of blood to the injured hand while the body brings its own clotting mechanisms to bear.

Living Things

Classification of Living Things

The study of living things begins with the system by which living things are classified. There are two major divisions and many lesser divisions involved in classifying living organisms. An understanding of the classification system used to describe and to order living things is useful for the prenursing student. After entering into nursing study, you will be called upon to use such things as genus-species nomenclature when referring to common illness-producing microorganisms such as *Haemophilus influenza*, which causes the flu, or *Vibrio comma*, which causes cholera. A traditional way of looking at living things involves separating the universe of living things into the plant and the animal kingdoms and then moving down the line into smaller and smaller divisions. Classification proceeds thus:

Kingdom	Animal or Plant
Phylum and Subphylum	Division culminates in Vertebrates (animals with a spinal cord) or Invertebrates (animals without a spinal cord).
Class	Vertebrates are divided into Pisces (fish), Amphibians (water- and land-dwelling animals), Reptiles, Avians (birds), and Mammals.
Order	Among animals, involves such things as whether the creature was meat-eating or vegetarian.
Family	A major subdivision, such as cat, dog, or bat.
Genus	Almost at the end! Capitalized Latin name, such as *Homo*, in the case of a human, or *Canus*, in the case of a dog.
Species	Final, noncapitalized name, which appears following the genus name for final identification, as in *Homo sapiens*.

Nursing students may find many of the genus and species identifiers used in the health care world familiar. For example, the modern world has become quite familiar with the term *E. coli*, which is the genus and species name abbreviation for *Eschericia coli*. This culprit causes disease in the case of contaminated beef products, such as hamburger. Examples of other microorganisms capable of producing disease in humans are *Mycobacterium tuberculae*, the organism producing tuberculosis, or *Staphylococcus aureus*, a famous offender for those who become hospital patients.

Among these simple organisms, there is a major division at the animal and plant kingdom level: protozoa (small animal disease-producers), bacteria (plant kingdom microbes), and viruses. In terms of classification, viruses are in a special category all their own. They exhibit different behaviors from the other two types of small organisms known to affect humans and other mammals. Most importantly, they are not affected by antimicrobial substances, such as penicillin, or the arsenicals used to kill parasites. The bacteria are those microbes that will be killed by use of antibiotics. The protozoa or even more complex animal-kingdom creatures that infest humans can be killed by smaller doses of what would kill humans, such as arsenic compounds. This provides a partial explanation as to why not all infections can be cured through antibiotic use or by things that would kill human parasites.

As you review, you will develop an understanding of such relationships.

Practice with Science Questions

Directions: Review the material on the classification of living things and then answer the following questions.

1. The lowest, or final, term on the classfication list for living things is

    (A) phylum.
    (B) class.
    (C) species.
    (D) order.

2. The two kingdoms by which living things are classified are

    (A) genus and species.
    (B) phylum and order.
    (C) organic and inorganic.
    (D) plant and animal.

3. A likely genus and species name would be

    (A) *Onomatopeia.*
    (B) *Clostridium difficile.*
    (C) *Canus, major.*
    (D) *Serratia Alfredo.*

Answers:

1. **(C)** The order would be kingdom, phylum, class, order, family, genus, and species. Therefore, the final term in the list would be species.

2. **(D)** The two kingdoms are plant and animal.

3. **(B)** For a correct genus and species name, there should be a capitalized first Latin term followed by an uncapitalized second term. Choice B is the only one that follows these rules. Choice A has only one term. Choice C involves a comma inserted between the two terms. Choice D capitalizes both terms.

Concepts of Organic Chemistry

ATOMS, ELEMENTS, AND MOLECULES

Just as there is an orderly way in which to classify living organisms, substances out of which living things are built can also be categorized. The usual categorization system involves size and other descriptive properties. The smallest things in terms of size are atoms, although scientists speculate that there are building blocks, given such colorful names as quarks and leptons, for even such infinitesimally small things as the parts of the atom. The atom consists of the nucleus, containing a certain number of neutrons and protons. Circling around the nucleus will be an electron shell or shells. Each substance has a different number of all these particles. Neutrons and protons, housed within the nucleus, or center, of the atom, are said to weigh something. They give the atom its mass. In addition, protons are said to loosely attract electrons in such a way that a ring of almost-weightless electrons circulates around the nucleus, much as moons cruise around a planet. It is important to understand that, when an electron's outer shell is incompletely filled, it will forever be ready to share an outer electron shell with another nearby atom.

From such small beginnings, life arises. The basic 118 elements are made up of atoms of the same type. For example, sodium is a basic type of atom, otherwise called an element. When these sodium atoms get together with another type of element's atoms, they form molecules, out of which life is born and sustained. When the element sodium combines with chloride, common table salt is formed. Water is formed when the element (or atom) called hydrogen gets together with the element (or atom) called oxygen. Water is made up of *atoms* of hydrogen and atoms of oxygen. Put another way, water is made up of the *elements* hydrogen and oxygen. Atoms make up the elements: the simplest types of matter. When more than one of these types of atom or element combine by sharing an outer electron shell, or ring, they become molecules. Water is both a molecule and a compound. When molecules are in the same general vicinity, they are visible to the human eye as such things as table salt or water or ammonia.

As you can see, things are never as simple as they seem on the surface. Batches of molecules, or compounds, are usually visible, but these substances are not always visible. Compounds can exist as solid substances, which are visible, of course, and some compounds may exist as liquids at room temperature, which are normally visible. However, a compound may exist as a gas, which may be either visible or invisible to the human eye. This property of being solid, liquid, or gas is called the state of the compound, or the state of matter.

Returning to the subject of elements, certain elements are so important to internal human function that, among hospitalized patients, tests are run on an almost-daily basis to detect levels of these within the human bloodstream. One of the most common serum chemistry tests examines a blood sample for presence of the elements sodium, potassium, chloride, magnesium, and calcium. In order to recognize these test results, you should learn the chemical symbols taken directly from the Periodic Table of the Elements: Na, K, Cl, Mg, and Ca. In the test results, small plus or minus signs usually accompany these symbols.

Practice with Science Questions

Directions: Review the material on organic chemistry and then answer the following questions.

1. Which are the smallest particles of matter?

   (A) atoms
   (B) molecules
   (C) substances
   (D) compounds

2. Basic elements are made up of individual

   (A) molecules.
   (B) moles.
   (C) atoms.
   (D) compounds.

3. Approximately how many basic elements have been discovered?

   (A) 11
   (B) 118
   (C) 211
   (D) 55

4. The particle of the atom that forms bonds with other atoms by sharing an outer shell, or ring, is the

   (A) neutron.
   (B) proton.
   (C) electron.
   (D) neutrino.

5. An atom is to _____ as a molecule is to a compound.

   (A) fission
   (B) a substance
   (C) an ion
   (D) an element

6. The three states of matter are

   (A) ions, molecules, and compounds.
   (B) solid, liquid, and gas.
   (C) frozen, boiling, and airborne.
   (D) inert, active, and encapsulated.

Answers:

1. **(A)** Atoms are the smallest particles of matter.

2. **(C)** Atoms make up elements.

3. **(B)** 118.

4. **(C)** Electrons bond and are located in the outer ring.

5. **(D)** An atom is to an *element* as a molecule is to a compound.

6. **(B)** The three states are *solid, liquid,* and *gas.*

We need to review several additional concepts from the field of organic chemisty. These are ionization, acid-base concepts, and aerobic and anaerobic metabolism.

IONIZATION

As just noted, elements such as sodium, potassium, chloride, magnesium, and calcium are important to internal human function. When these elements are found outside the body, they appear in dry form in combination with other elements. Sodium chloride (NaCl), or table salt, is a good example. When some compounds, such as table salt, are placed into a liquid, usually a water-based substance, they dissolve into their constituent elements again. Table salt forms sodium ions and chloride ions. These ions possess a charge, either positive or negative. The charge will cause them to be reattracted to their oppositely charged "mate" when the liquid evaporates. An ion, therefore, is an electrically charged atom. (Electrically charged atoms may carry a positive charge when dissolved [cation] or a negative charge [anion].)

For example, sodium is a cation and possesses a positive charge and will, therefore, should the water evaporate, be attracted to the negatively charged anion, chloride, once again. In dry form, cations, with their positive charge, will link with anions, with their negative charge, to re-form molecules, or compounds. In the case of the water that evaporates, it would leave a salt residue behind.

In the human body, elements appear in their ion form, floating within the liquid areas of the body—the bloodstream (vascular spaces), the body's individual cells (intracellular spaces), and the spaces surrounding the cells (extracellular spaces). The human body prefers that a steady state consisting of an exact range of these elements be maintained. Whenever an element rises toward too high a level, built-in mechanisms ensure that the preferred range is maintained. A severe excess of any of these elements will result in the death of the organism. The same thing is true of preferred body temperature ranges and acid-base ranges. Built-in control mechanisms within land-dwelling organisms also ensure that a comfortable zone of temperature and acid-base balance is maintained.

ACID-BASE PRINCIPLES

Acid-base is expressed using the term pH. The pH of a substance is expressed as a number within the range 0 to 14. When discussing pH, we usually think of liquid substances. If we wanted to influence the pH of a neutral substance, having a pH of 7, such as plain water, we would add either an acid or an alkaline (base) substance. If we added lemon juice, a mildly acidic substance, to a glass of water (pH 7), the pH would drop, as the substance became more acidic. The pH might drop slightly to 6.5 or so with the addition of a little bit of the weak acid. Even with the addition of a large amount of the weak acid, the pH might drop no lower than 6. But if we poured in a very strong acid, such as hydrochloric acid (pH approximately 1.0), the glass of water's pH would drop dramatically. Do not mix water and hydrochloric acid at home because it could cause a rather strong and unexpected reaction. From this brief discussion, you can see that an acid solution has a pH of less than 7.0, whereas a neutral substance has a pH of 7.0. The body prefers that the pH remain within a narrow range within the center of the pH scale, becoming neither too acidic nor too alkaline.

Now, if we wanted to influence a plain glass of water to become more basic, or alkaline, we would need to add a base, such as ammonium hydroxide. After adding a small amount of the ammonium hydroxide, the resultant strong-smelling mixture would have a pH of 8 or 9, which is mildly basic.

The human body prefers that the internal pH range, within the bloodstream, remain within, roughly speaking, the area of 7.35 to 7.45. Anything that falls very far outside this range will not support life. When the internal environment falls below pH 7.0 or above the alkaline state of 7.9, this is considered to be a panic situation. Even though certain individual compartments, such as the stomach cavity, can tolerate extremes, the cells, intracellular spaces, and vascular compartments prefer something that approaches a more neutral state.

Practice with Science Questions

Directions: Review the material on substances in solution and then answer the following questions.

1. Which of the following is a positively charged cation?

(A) potassium
(B) hydroxide
(C) chloride
(D) hydroxyl

2. If you knew that the normal level of potassium in the bloodstream of a human was 3.5 to 5.0, what would you expect to happen should the potassium level rise to 7.0?

   (A) The results are impossible to predict.
   (B) Nothing, the body is very efficient at handling extremes.
   (C) The person would die.
   (D) None of the above. Humans do not have potassium in their bloodstreams.

3. A solution with a pH of 9.0 is

   (A) acid.
   (B) alkaline.
   (C) neutral.
   (D) a cation.

4. A solution with a pH of 2.0 is

   (A) acid.
   (B) alkaline.
   (C) neutral.
   (D) a cation.

5. If a solution had a pH of 7.0 and one added a solution with a pH of 6.0, the resulting solution becomes

   (A) more acidic.
   (B) more alkaline.
   (C) a colloid.
   (D) neutral.

6. The human body prefers to be

   (A) acidic.
   (B) alkaline.
   (C) approximately neutral.
   (D) none of the above.

Answers:

1. **(A)** Potassium is a cation.

2. **(C)** Very high or very low levels of ions are incompatible with life.

3. **(B)** It would be alkaline.

4. **(A)** It would be acid.

5. **(A)** It would be more acidic.

6. **(C)** The human body prefers to be approximately neutral.

AEROBIC AND ANAEROBIC METABOLISM

There are two final foundational concepts involving the internal environment of living things—metabolism in the presence of a rich supply of oxygen (aerobic, or with oxygen) and metabolism in the absence of oxygen (anaerobic, or without oxygen). Metabolism produces energy for survival and involves the cell's ability to produce energy from the basic nutrients of carbohydrates, fats, and proteins. Every moment that a cell lives, it is manipulating these substances, in the presence of oxygen or, temporarily, in its absence, to produce energy for survival.

Glucose is the substance that is most often manipulated to produce energy, but fat or protein substances may also be used. In humans, aerobic metabolism is the preferred mode, but anaerobic may be used in its absence. In fact, humans and other creatures often have back-up mechanisms. The anaerobic process is not as efficient, but it is used routinely. For example, the muscle cells of a runner who cannot take in enough oxygen to supply heavily working muscles in the middle of a run rely on anaerobic metabolism. Another case of anaerobic metabolism that is important to nurses is the code situation, wherein the person's breathing pattern is erratic at best, insufficient oxygen is taken in, and the muscles and other cells are forced to revert to the back-up mechanism—anaerobic metabolism. To compound the problem, the heart cannot pump sufficient oxygen around in the bloodstream to transport it to the cells that need it, so, once again, cells are forced to work in the absence of their usual rich supply of oxygen.

Remember that the anaerobic form of metabolism in mammals is less efficient than the aerobic form because anaerobic metabolism cannot be maintained forever. It produces only about 5 or 6 percent (1/20th) of the energy produced by aerobic metabolism. It is designed to be temporary.

Anaerobic metabolism also produces byproducts that will affect the overall acid-base balance of the body adversely. Normally, the cells use oxygen and nutrients (glucose, protein, and fat substances) to produce energy and to produce two major byproducts—water and carbon dioxide. The byproduct carbon dioxide is efficiently removed from the body through the normal breathing mechanism. Were it to linger within the body, an acidic state would tend to occur. The byproducts of anaerobic metabolism are not as easily handled. In the case of the skeletal muscles, lactic acid is the byproduct of anaerobic metabolism. Too much lactic acid will, in time, overwhelm the body's buffering and excretion mechanisms.

Practice with Science Questions

1. What are factors that influence the body to become more acidic when breathing and heartbeat stop, as in an emergency situation?

   (A) Anaerobic metabolism (lactic acid production).
   (B) Carbon dioxide is not transported to the lungs.
   (C) Carbon dioxide is not exhaled out of the body.
   (D) All of the above.

2. Which of the following may be used by the body to produce energy?

   (A) Glucose, fat, and oxygen.
   (B) Ammonia and carbon dioxide.
   (C) Cellulose and bicarbonate.
   (D) None of the above.

Answers:

   1. **(D)**

   2. **(A)**

Cells and Simple Organisms

In the normal course of events, certain necessary conditions must exist for life to endure. One condition involves the fact that living cells must almost always be bathed in a liquid medium, or at least one that is no more solid than a type of jelly. Whether one considers the size or complexity of the organism, individual cells need to live within a nutrient medium. Each cell must be bathed continually and must have access to exchange mechanisms within this liquid or gelatinous home in which it survives. According to an old saying, when creatures first left the oceans, they had to be sophisticated enough to have transferred the salty, mineral-rich, sealike environment into their internal structure. Because these new land-dwellers could no longer float around in sea water, they needed to have internal pathways through which the sea water could bathe and feed the individual cells. In humans and the other mammals, this is done efficiently through a complex internal clustering of tissues and transport systems.

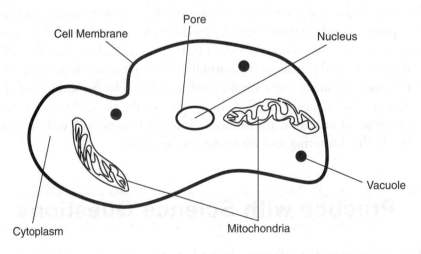

The Cell

Picture the individual cells of any living thing. These cells have an outer wall that acts as a barrier to things that the cell does not need at any given time. This wall is called the cell membrane. In some of the smaller organisms, under conditions of stress, the cell membrane can even help to protect the organism by forming itself into a type of shield, called a spore. The cell also has an internal medium, termed protoplasm or cytoplasm, consisting of liquid or gel with dissolved substances in it.

Within the protoplasm, the cell usually has energy storage or transfer bodies, called vacuoles. They help out when the cell needs something that is not readily available or is complex to produce. Mitochondria within the cytoplasm assist with production and release of energy. The cell has a center area, or nucleus, that contains coding for reproducing either internal substances on demand, the ribonucleic acid (RNA) system, or the entire cell when conditions dictate that it is the correct time, the deoxyribonucleic acid (DNA) system.

With this equipment, the cell must be able to

1. Take in nutrients, typically by diffusion through the cell wall or membrane;
2. Take in either oxygen (animals) or carbon dioxide (plants);
3. Excrete waste products or byproducts of metabolism (water and carbon dioxide, in the case of animals);
4. Synthesize, or form more complex things from simple things, producing or releasing energy in the process;
5. Regulate the internal environment (pH and temperature);
6. Move, in some fashion, or have an internal medium that permits movement of substances from point to point; and
7. Reproduce.

DIFFUSION AND OSMOSIS

Let us pause briefly to consider how the cell absorbs what it needs and disposes of what it does not need. This is done through diffusion and osmosis.

Diffusion is the passage of substances from an area of higher concentration to an area of lower concentration. It can occur in a gas, such as air, or a liquid, such as water. If you sprayed perfume in a room, you would see diffusion in action. The perfume will soon spread throughout the air of the room, which originally held a low concentration of perfume, and you will be able to smell the fragrance anywhere within the room.

With liquid media, diffusion involves the passage of substances *in solution* from an area of higher concentration to an area of lower concentration. To see diffusion in a liquid medium, mix a little bit of food coloring with some table salt, place the colored table salt in a napkin or cloth of some sort, and then submerge the napkin full of green salt in a bowl of water. The colored salt will leach out into the bowl of water, making it a paler, but still ugly, shade of green. To pass into the bowl of water, the salt first must dissolve in the water that entered the napkin and then, still existing within the napkin, head for the area of lower green-salt concentration, the water in the bowl. The diffusion process stops when the concentration in the bowl reaches the concentration within the submerged napkin. Try this experiment on your own. You could also break off a plant stem and submerge it in a cup of water tinted with dark blue food coloring. After a day or two, the leaf at the top will turn blue, resembling the messier green-salt diffusion experiment.

Within living things, the process of diffusion explains how such substances as potassium or sodium can pass into individual cells. Depending on the strength of the concentration, potassium or any other ion will simply diffuse very quietly through the cell membrane.

Osmosis is a slightly more complex process by which liquids are drawn toward such complex molecules as colloids. You must picture colloids as being like jelly or a pasty substance when dry, rather than a salt, if you are to form a mental image of osmosis. Semipermeable membranes are involved in osmosis because they do not permit the passage of colloids, the more complex molecules that tend to attract liquids.

The human bloodstream provides an example of osmosis. When blood courses through the network of blood vessels within the human body, osmosis guards against all of humanity resembling balloonlike creatures. With each beat of our hearts, blood is forcefully pumped out and enters a network of blood vessels. Due to pressure from within blood vessels during this forceful pumping action, some of the liquid portion of blood leaks out into the interstitial areas (the stuff in which the cells live). However, more liquid leaves the blood vessels than is taken in and used by cells, so there is a net loss to the intravascular space (the part within the blood vessels). If nothing happened to ensure that liquid would reenter the bloodstream at the return-to-the-heart end of things, we would all begin to become puffier and puffier.

Tissues, Organs, Systems, Organisms

As we start to review how cells are organized into more complex things, we will look at animal cells exclusively. With some exceptions, the plant kingdom operates in much the same way as the animal kingdom. These exceptions are not critical to your review for nursing entrance test purposes.

TISSUES

Cells of similar purpose tend to form into groups that become clustered together to perform a task; these are called tissues. Examples of tissues in humans and other animals would be the muscles, bones, or lining along the walls of the gastrointestinal tract. A fuller description of the types of mammalian tissues follows.

Epithelial Tissue

Epithelial tissue covers the body and lines surfaces of areas that communicate with the outside world. It serves a protective function, in that it lines the gastrointestinal tract, the respiratory system, blood vessels, and the reproductive and urinary systems. Epithelial cells can be of the squamous variety (flat), columnar, or ciliated. One specialized function of epithelial tissues is ciliary action, the movement of mucus and particles upward out of the main respiratory tube system. Cilia resemble tiny hairs and tend to move from deeper to outer respiratory areas. Another specialized function of epithelial tissue is secretion, such as mucus or endocrine (glandular) substances. Mucus keeps tissues moist, whereas glandular secretions can be thought of as messenger substances, designed to extend the range of the nervous, or control, system throughout the body. But epithelial cells also perform a more direct neurologic function, sensing things coming into the body, such as with taste or smell.

When compared with certain other specialized tissue, epithelial tissue can repair itself quickly. The cells rapidly reproduce throughout the lifespan of the organism. It is a simple sort of tissue and may be thought of as one of the most primitive.

Connective Tissue

If epithelial tissue can be thought of as a thin and simple covering that protects large areas of the body, connective tissue can be thought of as a structural, shape-associated tissue. In humans, connective tissue makes up bone and cartilage. In more primitive creatures, such as certain types of sea creatures, connective tissue forms an outer shell.

Connective tissue gives an organism its shape, making it recognizable. Connective tissue also serves to protect the body from physical trauma or assault. Connective tissue forms a sort of carapace over and around the human chest cavity, protecting the vitally necessary heart and lungs from damage. It does the same with the dense and compact bony covering of the spine and of the cranium, which houses the brain.

In addition to the hard, boney protective coverings, connective tissue is also found in the body's nutrient storage systems; fatty tissue is a type of connective tissue. Although fatty tissues are primarily used as a food storage system by animals that hibernate in winter, it also carries humans through times of problems with access to food supplies.

The elastic arterial tissue of some of the blood vessels and the cartilaginous tissue of, say, the nose are also made of connective tissue. Ligaments and tendons, those bands of tissue that connect muscle to bone, are also connective. It could be said that connective tissue is characterized by strength, structural connectivity, and some degree of elasticity.

Reproductive Tissue

Reproductive tissue for a particular organism carries genetic coding. The tissue is specialized in a very particular way. It is the only tissue in the body that will not divide until separated programming, or genetic coding, is brought together, into close proximity. Following a brief introduction here, additional information on the history of the study of genetics and problems with genetic coding in humans will appear in a later section.

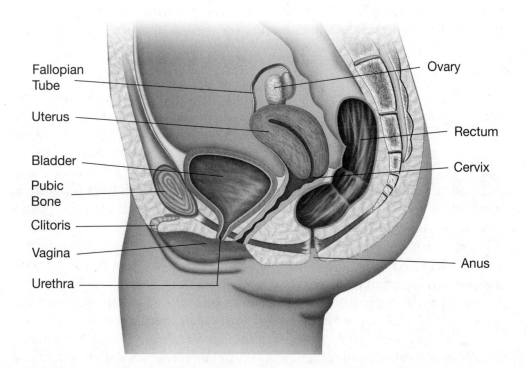

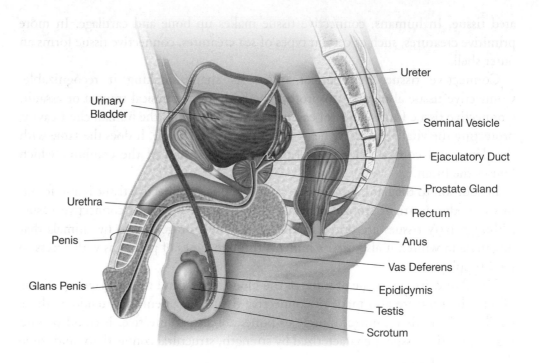

In mammals, including humans, sperm cells contain the genetic code contributed by the male of the species, while egg cells, which are destined to remain within the female until the birth of a new organism, contribute the other part of the genetic code. Females are born with all the egg cells they will ever have, whereas, within the male, sperm cells may be formed closer to time of use.

When the two types of cells unite, a new creature will begin to be formed. The initial germ, or germination, cells will differentiate into the many types of tissues that represent all those tissues that will be needed by the new creature, according to a pre-set timing program contained within the original genetic material. If internal conditions are maintained at an acceptable level within the female mammal, this new creature will emerge into the outside world after a period of growth, or gestation.

Blood

Just as certain secretions, such as those of glandular tissues, have a communicative function, so do blood cells and the system that supports them. Blood cells arise from the marrow located in the center areas of certain bones, such as the sternum (breastbone), iliac crests (part of the hip/pelvic structure), and the long leg bones (femurs). Blood cells are primitive at first and do not differentiate into their three mature types until ready to enter the bloodstream, the liquid portion of which is termed plasma. Occasionally, under various conditions of stress, blood cells will enter the plasma before they mature. This can be a useful diagnostic factor in relation to some diseases.

The three types of mature blood cells are red cells, white cells, and platelets. Red blood cells carry hemoglobin, which binds with oxygen at the lung area of the body. The oxygen is carried throughout the body with each beat of the heart. White blood cells are responsible for handling microorganisms or other foreign, organic matter that enters the body. Their job is one of defense. Platelets are associated with clotting.

The fact that these cells are produced in the interior of strong and protected areas of the body bespeaks their importance to human life. Like epithelial cells, the blood cells are rapidly forming, fast-growing cells. Consequently, they are vulnerable to assault by certain chemical or biological agents, as well as being susceptible to the effects of ionizing radiation.

Muscle Tissue

One of the functions of living things is movement. Among the higher forms of water-dwelling creatures, muscle tissue is essential to those that engage in active forms of nutrient procurement. The same is true of nonmicroscopic land-dwelling creatures.

Providing a means for locomotion, muscles attach to bones and, through a series of sophisticated stretching and relaxation maneuvers, allow creatures to move about the surface of the planet or the depths of the ocean. Voluntary muscle tissue attaches to bones for the purpose of gross or fine motor activity. It responds to our desire to move. Muscle tissue also forms cardiac tissue, a specialized type of tissue involved with heart activity. A third type of specialized muscle tissue, smooth muscle, moves substances through the gastrointestinal tract and is involved with the elasticity of certain blood vessels. Smooth muscle is an involuntary muscle tissue in that it responds to internal and unconscious control mechanisms.

Nerve Tissue

As the master control system for voluntary acts, nerve tissue serves several vital purposes. It is responsible for receiving information about the outside environment and for communicating this information. If we consider the endocrine system to be an extension of nerve tissue, then it also regulates internal systems. This internal regulation involves maintaining a steady internal temperature or preferentially shunting blood to certain areas during times of stress.

Nerve tissue can be either peripheral or central, sensory or motor. The mechanisms involved with these types of internal communication are discussed in the next section on organs and systems.

ORGANS AND SYSTEMS

Tissues of a certain type cluster together to form organs. Organs, in turn, are grouped together according to tissue type and overall function. Depending on the classification method used, there are anywhere from five to ten organ systems in mammals.

You should be familiar with the following systems:

1. Neuroendocrine
2. Musculoskeletal
3. Gastrointestinal
4. Cardiorespiratory
5. Renal/urinary
6. Reproductive
7. Integumentary

The Neuroendocrine System

The neuroendocrine system is composed of the nervous system and the endocrine system. Even though both component systems send and receive messages by exchanging chemicals, the nervous system's activities rely on sets of pathways and a rapid pace of action. By contrast, the endocrine system is more ubiquitous: its chemicals are "ductless" and tend to travel throughout certain body regions without the need for established, relatively linear pathways.

The nervous system consists of the central nervous system (CNS), which encompasses the brain and spinal cord, and the peripheral nervous system (PNS), which extends out to internal organs, hands, feet, and almost all other areas of the body. The nervous system consists of afferent and efferent nerves. Afferent nerves carry impulses from various areas of the body to the spinal cord and/or brain and are responsible for recognition related to touch, pressure, seeing, hearing, and the like. Afferent nerves are also called sensory nerves. In contrast, efferent nerves carry impulses from the central nervous system out to the periphery or to internal organs, such as the heart or the stomach. These are often called motor nerves, or motor neurons. They are responsible for movement, either of the organism as a whole or of selected parts of the organism.

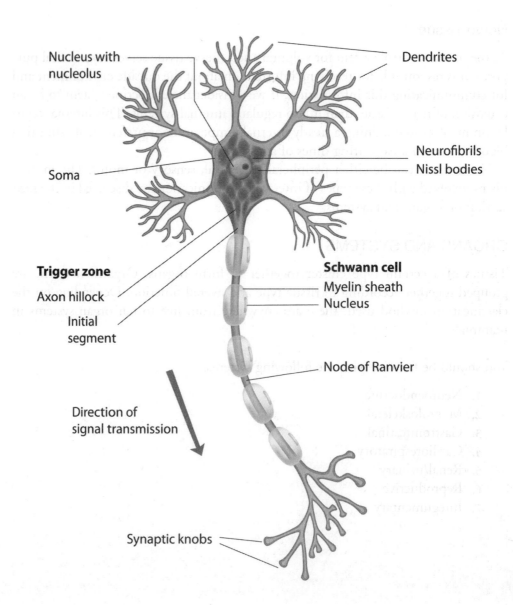

Science Review   **221**

This network of nerves runs throughout the body. Nerve-to-nerve communication is effected by means of transmitter substances that travel forward, are received by special receptor areas, and then are deactivated and/or returned to their point of origin. The available levels of these substances or the amounts that remain after activation are thought to play a role in such difficult-to-pinpoint areas as mood, memory, or perceived energy levels.

Although parts of the central nervous system are unable to grow again when damaged, bony casings such as the spinal column and the cranium generally protect this area. In addition, the medulla, which is a carefully protected area of the brain, regulates breathing and heartbeat. The lungs and the heart often continue to function even in the event of severe brain damage.

The peripheral nervous system is made up of the somatic and the autonomic divisions. The somatic division of the PNS involves nerve impulses to and from skeletal muscles and is thought to be under the individual's control. When we tell something to move, it does. This is a result of adequate somatic nervous system function.

On the other hand, the autonomic division helps control the internal organs and is considered to be largely involuntary. It reacts in certain ways without conscious direction on the part of the organism. It operates during periods of both sleep and wakefulness. The autonomic division, in turn, is divided into the sympathetic and parasympathetic nervous systems.

The sympathetic system is often called the fight-or-flight system because it is activated in times of stress and is responsible for mustering the energy, speed, and keen reactions needed in a crisis.

Basically speaking, the parasympathetic nervous system is the system that is predominant in normal times and that takes over once a crisis or stress situation has passed.

The master nerve centers of the neuroendocrine system are the thalamus and its extension, the hypothalamus. Both organs lie close to and communicate with the pituitary gland. All are seated in a highly protected and centrally located area of the brain. The pituitary gland is known as the master gland in that it controls the activities of other glands. Its divisions are the anterior pituitary and posterior pituitary. The posterior pituitary secretes the antidiuretic hormone, which is responsible for making the body retain fluid in time of threat or low levels of fluid. The posterior pituitary also secretes pitressin/oxytocin, which stimulates uterine contractions as a part of the birth process. It can be seen why, with involvement in both survival and reproduction, this gland is of vital interest to mammalian organisms.

The anterior part of the pituitary also plays an important role in survival. Through adrenocorticotropic hormone (ACTH), it stimulates the adrenal cortex areas, located at the kidneys, to secrete certain vital hormones such as cortisone, a steroid. Cortisone plays a role in internal fluid balance and in muscle maintenance and energy levels. The middle parts of the adrenal glands are also important in survival. The medulla produces adrenaline, or epinephrine, which helps the body muster internal energy stores, such as sugars, and creates a sequence of events designed to maintain the body's ability to respond to threat. Adrenaline is the body's fight-or-flight hormone. As part of the individual's reaction under threat, the adrenal medulla's activities are to maintain blood pressure and to stave off shock and the immediate effects of trauma. The air passages are opened (bronchodilation), and the heart beats faster and more forcefully. The pupils of the eye dilate and distance vision is improved. Clotting will be more rapid. Circulation to areas of digestion is lessened, whereas circulation to skeletal muscle is fostered.

Although cortisone and adrenaline are useful in typical internal quantities, there are problems when steroids are taken into the body in larger quantities. This is also thought to be one of the problems with chronic steroid use. Not only does it lead to the lessening of inflammatory responses over time and the building of muscle groups, particularly when used by athletes who are actively training, but it also may be addictive. The individual may come to rely on the mood-elevating properties of this sort of substance.

Another anterior pituitary hormone, growth hormone, is involved with the regulation of what could be thought of as one of the many biological clocks. This particular clock causes overall musculoskeletal growth to occur more rapidly at some times and less rapidly at others. Without proper functioning in relation to the growth hormone, adult humans tend to be too big or too small in comparison with other humans.

The anterior pituitary also secretes the thyroid-stimulating hormone. This hormone stimulates the thyroid gland, located at the front of the neck, to maintain or alter the metabolic rate of internal processes. Other glands located nearby, the parathyroids, are involved with activities of some of the body's basic minerals, such as calcium.

Two other anterior pituitary hormones are responsible for milk production by mothers, and for reproductive function in both males and females. Both of these activities are equally necessary for survival of the species.

Through hormonal systems, organisms can initiate survival mechanisms in times of threat. They can also return to a state of average function when external or internal threat abates. Through this complex system of receiving signals, reacting, with or without conscious thought, and controlling the internal environment before, during, and after stimuli are received, the body maintains economy of effort as well as a capacity to react to save itself.

The Musculoskeletal System

One of the more important body systems in relation to the ability of the animal kingdom's creatures to respond to various needs is the musculoskeletal system. Plants, in general, do not possess the ability to move about at will, but members of the animal kingdom, whether fish in the sea or land-dwelling creatures, are in almost constant motion, whether searching for things or simply moving about out of habit. This tendency to move about is also important when it is necessary to escape from threat. The musculoskeletal system is useful not only in moving, but also in protecting internal organs.

The ribs protect the heart and lungs, which are vital to the on-going need to deliver cellular supplies and remove cellular wastes. Without heart and lung function, the cells of the body will die within minutes. Protection from external damage is needed over the chest area.

The pelvic bones protect reproductive areas, as well as certain nerve trunks that pass through on their way to the legs. Leg function is also important in the body's need to escape or to seek. Without legs, land animals would not be able to live very long in the wild.

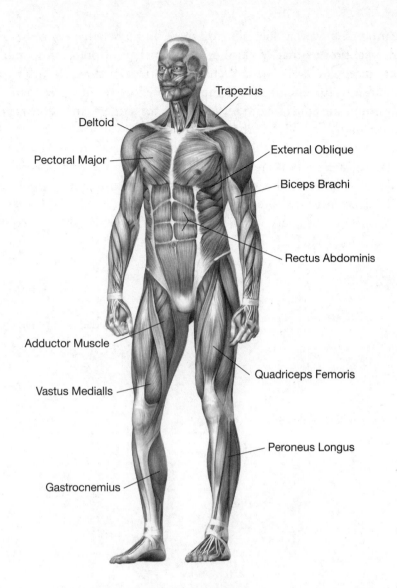

Trapezius
Deltoid
Pectoral Major
External Oblique
Biceps Brachi
Rectus Abdominis
Adductor Muscle
Quadriceps Femoris
Vastus Medialls
Peroneus Longus
Gastrocnemius

Finally, the bones and muscles of the arms and legs are the components of loco-motion. When combined with sophisticated neurosensory components, they fulfill living creatures' needs to move about the surface of the earth, to bring things close to sensory intake and nutrient intake areas, and to learn. The musculoskeletal system makes us an evolving group, contributing to our capacity to be sentient, self-aware beings.

The Gastrointestinal System

Two divisions are involved with getting nutrients ready to be delivered at the cellular level. The first arises when nutrients are taken into the food tube, our gastrointestinal system, worked upon by food tube processes, and allowed to linger in the intestines at the interface between the food tube and internal circulation. The function of this first division is similar to what a flatworm does as it sifts dirt and nutrients into its gullet, processes these for absorption into internal tissues, and, finally, eliminates the plain, nonuseful dirt from its little system. In humans and other higher-than-worm creatures, the food tube mechanisms culminate in absorption of the broken-down molecules of nutrients for absorption into the bloodstream and the elimination from the gut of leftover material.

The process, however, does not stop there. In higher-than-worm creatures, there is an internal process that constitutes the latter half of preparation and delivery of nutrients at cellular level. The molecules of nutrients pass across the intestinal membranes and into the circulation. Some are stored in various predesignated areas of the body, some are converted to related forms for storage, and some are delivered to cells throughout the body via the bloodstream.

Certain types of external substances will be absorbed and used by the body's cells, and those substances that are not useful will be eliminated from the gut without ever having been absorbed beyond the intestine's membranous barrier. In simplified form, the substances that are useful and that are absorbed into the circulation are proteins, carbohydrates, fats, water, vitamins, and minerals. All can be obtained from recognizable food sources.

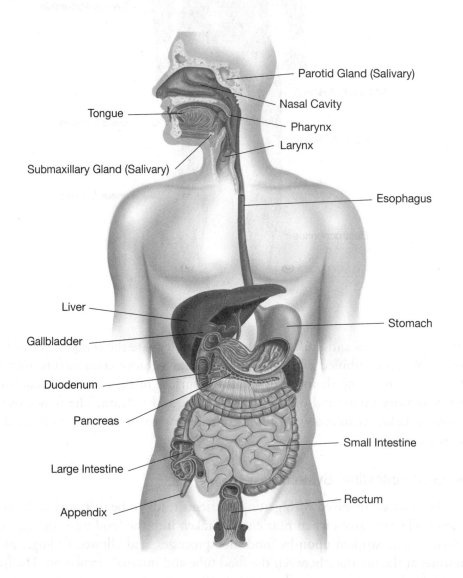

As food is taken into the mouth, some is chewed by the teeth, mechanically breaking down the larger pieces. In addition, saliva, which contains the enzyme ptyalin, works to break down complex carbohydrates into simpler structures. Next, the food is swallowed, passing through the epiglottis into the esophagus, the food tube area at the back of the throat. This cartilaginous, ringed food tube propels the food downward, through the cardiac sphincter, and into the stomach. The cardiac sphincter is a most important anatomic structure. It allows food to pass into the heavily acidic medium of the stomach, without allowing food, acids, or acidic gases to linger at the distal end (far portion) of the esophagus. Nor must the cardiac sphincter allow reflux (backward passage) of such things after they enter the stomach. The cardiac sphincter is located at the delicate area of the diaphragm. If an individual is lucky, the cardiac sphincter will remain perfectly positioned at exactly that spot for a lifetime.

pH is one reason why it is so important that this sphincter be the gatekeeper to the stomach. When signaled to do so, the stomach fills with hydrochloric acid, a strong substance designed to break down more complex foods into simpler compounds. The stomach walls are lined with a special material and are protected from being digested by the acid. There is a base quality, or alkaline quality to this protection within the stomach. However, no such protection exists in the distal area of the esophagus should acid and food or acidic gases pass in reverse. The esophageal tissue will erode over time, giving rise to aches, a burning sensation, pain, and decreased enjoyment in eating. After years of such abuse, scar tissue may form, creating a narrowed opening into the stomach, with additional difficulties arising from the stricture's presence.

When the food in the stomach has been subjected to mechanical stomach churning and the action of acid and enzymes, it passes through the pyloric sphincter and into the first of three segments of the small intestine, the duodenum. Here, the substance is subjected to chemicals that enter through an inlet from the pancreas and the liver's bile duct. Bile, from the liver and the gallbladder, the liver's storage organ, helps break down fats into fatty acids and glycerol, forms in which fats may be absorbed into the bloodstream. Chemicals, or enzymes, from the pancreas help break down proteins into amino acids and carbohydrates into various forms of sugars, such as sucrose and glucose. All these substances will pass into the jejunum, the central part of the small intestine, for contact with the villi and absorption into the internal circulation. In the ileum, the final part of the small intestine, the liquid becomes slightly more solid as water is absorbed into the bloodstream. When this mushy substance passes into the large intestine, the work of absorption has been completed and it remains for the intestine to pass the now semisolid mass, along with its associated gases, through three sections of the large intestine and back out into the outside world.

In response to the absorption of the nutrients from a meal, the pancreas releases greater or lesser quantities of insulin to allow glucose to pass through cell walls and to be useful in the energy production process. While all this ingestion and digestion is going on, the regulatory areas of the body will shunt relatively greater quantities of blood to the organs of digestion and storage and relatively lesser quantities away from skeletal muscles and possibly, if it is felt to be safe, from the brain's cognitive and alertness need centers. The body is ready to relax after eating and, perhaps, to take a nap.

The Cardiorespiratory System

Carbohydrates, fats, proteins, minerals, vitamins, and water are the types of nutrients delivered to tissues. Additionally, tissues need an adequate supply of oxygen. But tissues also need a mechanism to transport nonneeded substances (liquids, solids, and gases) away from cells and to central exchange areas for clearance from the body. The cardiorespiratory system is the key mechanism by which all this is done.

To examine what happens when the cardiorespiratory system is functioning smoothly, let's start at the level of external respiration. Air enters the mouth and nose of land-dwelling creatures and passes through an airway system, known as the respiratory tree, to its eventual destination, the alveoli, located in the parenchyma (outermost spaces) of the lungs. The tree is made up of a large airway, known as the trachea, that bifurcates into the left mainstem bronchus and the right mainstem bronchus. The right mainstream bronchus is relatively straight, while the left curves to help create a pocket into which the heart will fit. These, in turn, become smaller, easily visible air passages, known as bronchi. The bronchi then turn into bronchioles. The bronchioles terminate in alveoli: little air sacs that resemble popcorn. The whole assembly resembles an upside-down elm tree, complete with the main trunk, the larger branches, the smaller branches, and, finally, the leaf sections. Without describing in detail how the air entering the lung is humidified and partially purified prior to arrival at the alveoli, let us just say that the entire air passage is designed to bring gases into contact at alveolar level, across a membrane, with the circulatory system. Gases are diffused across this alveolar-capillary membrane, which is the whole point of external respiration.

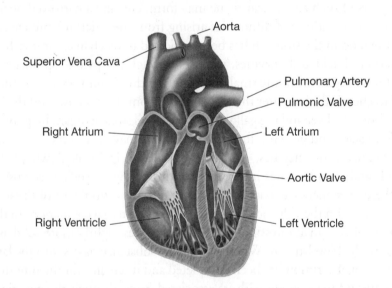

The system is so efficiently designed that muscle power is needed only to expand the rib cage and create a space into which air enters. This entering process is called inspiration. In the healthy creature, energy is not needed for the rib cage to return to its original shape, driving air out of the tree and exhausting gases into the outside world.

Humans have the additional ability, unlike any other creature, to communicate through speech. They can shape the larynx, or voice box, so that tissues allow for the utterance of distinct sounds as air passes into the lower areas of the tree. These sounds can be so carefully crafted that recognizable speech emerges to be captured and interpreted as symbols by other humans.

To understand what happens internally during respiration, we must consider the pump and the circulatory system, which work nonstop to deliver and eliminate substances at cellular level. The pump or heart is nestled between the right and left parts of the lung, carefully protected from the possibility of external damage. It has four chambers that facilitate the movement of blood through the heart. As blood returns from the body and brain, it enters the first of the heart's reception chambers, the right atrium. Blood entering this area is laden with carbon dioxide, a waste gas that is formed as a byproduct of cellular energy production. This blood is darker in color than the oxygen-rich blood at the other end of the system. From the right atrium, this blood travels into the second chamber, the right ventricle. From here, it passes through yet another one-way valve to the pulmonary artery and then to smaller vessels, known as arterioles, and finally on to the lung capillaries (the smallest of the lung's blood vessels) for gas diffusion. At the capillary level, the carbon dioxide passes out of the vessels, across the alveolar-capillary membrane, and into the respiratory tree for elimination during the expiratory phase of the process of external respiration. In turn, oxygen passes across the alveolar-capillary membrane from the alveoli and into the capillaries. Almost all the oxygen attaches to the hemoglobin found in the red blood cells and is swept along into venules, and then veins, and then one of the major four pulmonary veins, and finally back into the left atrium of the heart. This blood is oxygen-rich. It appears bright red as it passes through a powerful, one-way valve into the left ventricle, the most powerful chamber of the heart, for delivery to the body and brain. At this point, some of this oxygen-rich blood will be carried into the vessels that feed the all-important heart muscle tissue. The remainder will pass through other vessels to the brain and to the body.

As the blood makes its way to body and brain tissues, it passes through arteries into the smaller arterioles and then into capillaries. Along the way, a fair amount of liquid is forced out into the interstitium as the heart beats by hydrostatic pressure, the force of liquid against the walls of vessels. At the capillary level, nutrients and oxygen pass into the interstitium and then into cells by diffusion. Capillaries will become venules, then larger and larger veins as the blood returns to the heart. Some of the excess fluid remaining in the interstitium is drawn back into the venous blood supply by colloidal, or oncotic, pressure. The minute amount of liquid left behind at tissue level as this process occurs will generally be returned by the lymphatic system, a series of channels that are also important in infection control.

So far, we have examined the basics involved in the intake of oxygen and nutrients and their delivery to all the tissues of the body. We have examined the basics of gas elimination through the lung area and of solid waste elimination through the gastrointestinal system. What remains is an examination of the elimination of substances dissolved in liquid and of elimination of water itself from the body. The system that performs this is the urinary system. It is one of the most persistent and powerful regulators of internal balance. Without it, homeostasis would be impossible, and the organism would die.

The Renal/Urinary System

Located in the retroperitoneum, kidneys are a set of internal organs that are densely packed with capillaries and collecting ducts useful for bringing dissolved wastes into contact with a system of receptacles designed to carry waste out of the body. This excretion system is designed to eliminate exactly what is surplus while preserving liquids and dissolved substances necessary for meeting internal needs.

Within each kidney, little pockets of capillaries and collecting tubules form glomeruli. These come together to form larger tubules, which lead into the central collecting areas of the kidneys. Along the way, when capillaries and tubules are in proximity, substances pass out of the bloodstream, with internally needed substances being reabsorbed back into the bloodstream again at the distal (far) end of the tubules. In turn, tubules, which contain urine now, come together to form two ureters or long tubes, one to each half of the body, that allow urine to flow into the single bladder storage area. From this storage area, the urine flows through the urethra into the outside world.

Urine is made up of such things as water (over 90 percent), urea (a nitrogen product resulting from the breakdown of proteins), and various electrolytes (minerals). Typically, there should be no protein, sugar, or fat present in urine. Nor should there be any of the three types of blood cells. When any of these are present, the urinalysis is considered to be abnormal.

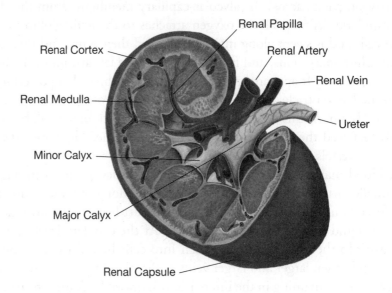

Maintaining internal acid-base balance is dependent on the renal/urinary sytem. Even though a specialized blood buffer system can return blood to a normal pH range in the face of an influx of acid or alkaline substances, it takes the combined power of lungs and kidneys to ensure lasting regulation of internal pH. Lungs work to eliminate acid by rapidly expelling carbon dioxide when an acidic state is pending. But lungs cannot eliminate enough carbon dioxide nor can they continue to eliminate it long enough to ensure regulation in the normal course of events. Therefore, one of the kidneys' most important functions is to allow urine to become relatively more acidic or more basic in response to the body's internal needs. It is the slowest but most powerful body system for regulating acid-base balance.

Genetics and Genomics

Sequencing denotes extracting the exact order of the bases or pairs in a strand of DNA. The identity of one base of a pair determines the other member base. The strand of DNA is treated with a variety of nucleotides (sets of enzymes) and a specific primer to generate a collection of smaller DNA fragments. The fragments include attached fluorescent tags. Fragments differ in length and size. The sequence is capable of being reconstructed by a computer. Today, researchers can use DNA sequencing to search for genetic variations and mutations that possibly relate in some way to the development of disease and illness.

The genome is an organism's complete set of DNA. Every cell in the body contains a complete copy of the approximately three billion DNA base pairs that make up the human genome. Genes carry information that makes all the proteins needed by organisms. These proteins determine the organism's appearance and behavior. Each gene (20,000–25,000) in the human genome codes for an average of three proteins.

Genes are located on 23 pairs of chromosomes that are attached to the nucleus of the human cell, and the genes direct the production of proteins with the assistance of enzymes and messenger molecules. The enzyme copies the information in a gene's DNA into a molecule called messenger ribonucleic acid RNA (mRNA). The mRNA travels out of the nucleus and into the cell's cytoplasm, where the mRNA is read by a tiny molecular machine called a ribosome, and the information is used to link together small molecules called amino acids in the correct order to form a specific protein. If a cell's DNA is mutated, it may produce an abnormal protein, which can disrupt the body's usual processes and lead to disease, such as cancer.

THE HUMAN GENOME PROJECT

The Human Genome Project (HGP) was originated in 1991 by the U.S. Department of Energy and the National Institutes of Health. It was completed in 2003. The project was a collaborative one with the original goal focused on the complete mapping and understanding of all the genes of human beings. The U.S. Department of Health and Human Services was renamed in 1997 to the National Human Genome Research Institute (NHGRI). Scientists across the world have access to this database. HGP researchers deciphered the human genome by determining the order of sequence of all the bases in the genome's DNA, making maps illustrating locations of genes for major sections of all chromosomes, and producing "linkage maps." In completing the HGP, the NHGRI are now able to include studies aimed at understanding how the human genome functions in the role of creating gene products, especially the numerous proteins for which genes code. The most recent quest in appreciating the human genome is in relation to the role it plays in both health and disease.

The world is fortunate to have genetic markers that are used for tracking inheritance of traits. Genetic mapping or "linkage mapping" is used first to isolate genes. With this information, criminal investigations and forensics are performed much more effectively and criminals are apprehended more efficiently. This mapping affirms evidence that a disease acquired from parent and linked to a child is because of the related genes. Genetic mapping was responsible for locating a single gene related to inherited diseases like muscular dystrophy. Genetic maps are known as microsatellite maps made using single-nucleotide polymorphisms or "snips" (SNPs). This process can map a disease or trait.

IMPLICATIONS OF GENOMICS FOR HEALTH CARE

Genetics and genome science are integrated into health care and are essential to the profession of nursing. As science and research continue to expand, new discoveries of managing diseases and illnesses will impact how care is delivered. It is imperative for nursing schools to incorporate genetics and genomics both didactically and clinically. For example, in the future, nursing will entail nurses knowing how to assist families specifically dealing with genetic issues and illnesses. Nurses will have acquired more knowledge about genetics and they will provide appropriate counseling to couples, rather than automatically referring them to a genetics counselor.

Genome.gov (2011) defines *genetics* as the study of individual genes and their impact on relatively rare single-gene disorders. *Genomics* is the study of all genes in the human genome together, including their interactions with each other and the environment and the influence of other psychosocial and cultural factors on them. Genetics and genomics will be applied at all levels of health care: promotion and prevention, screening, diagnosis, treatment selection, and evaluation. Advances in genome research linked to routine patient care will require intense research studies involving health care professionals. There are organizations, including the National Institutes of Health (NIH), Centers for Disease Control (CDC), American Nurses Association (ANA), and Oncology Nursing Society (ONS) to name a few, that support genomics and future discoveries.

CASE REVIEW: GENETIC NURSING

Hereditary Hemorrhagic Telangiectasia (HHT) genetically affects blood vessels of the body. One in 5,000 people are diagnosed with this horrific disease. Specific genetic findings involve family history (first-degree), abrupt and continuous nose bleeds, mucocultaneous telangiectases (small blanchable red spots at routine areas of the body, like legs, fingers, and nose), and visceral arteriovenous malformations (AVMs), most notably pulmonary, cerebral, gastrointestinal (GI), hepatic, spinal, or retinal. Nurses will acquire knowledge of this particular disease process in applying appropriate optimum care (Junglen et al., 2008).

In applying the nursing process, a thorough assessment would uncover data prior to actually examining the patient. Specific nursing diagnoses and planning are derived from identifying predetermined issues or needs of the patient. Treatment, education, care, and support are interventions instituted once testing has clinically confirmed appropriate genetic mutation. Identifying this mutation with one family member is sufficient without having other family members go through this process; others are diagnosed by providing a blood sample for testing (Junglen, et al., 2008).

There are programs designed to increase genetic literacy among the communities of people. But more has to be done creating and coordinating national programs designed specifically to enhance the public's understanding of the concepts of genetics and genomics as they relate to medicine.

HEREDITY AND REPRODUCTION. In discussing heredity, it is evident that higher organisms bring together the reproductive material, or genes, from two organisms. In the case of humans, a male and a female engage in sexual activity designed to unite a sperm cell with an egg cell. As is true with land-dwelling creatures in general, the male and female of the species have unique appearances and characteristics, designed to differentiate one from the other. These characteristics are also designed to attract.

There are 46 chromosomes, or gene carriers, in humans. The full human genetic code consists of thousands of gene sequences; this is also true of other creatures, such as birds or insects. These sequences are arranged in a complex fashion in chromosomes, present in the same numbers in all cells except the germ cells: the sperm and egg cells of land-dwelling, higher-order creatures. These specialized cells contain 44 complete chromosomes. But a final chromosome combination is possible only when a sperm unites with an egg. When this occurs among mammals, either a male or a female creature is formed. The male creature will have an X chromosome and a Y chromosome, so named from their configuration when viewed through a microscope. A female will have two X chromosomes. In addition to these gender-determining characteristics, the genes will determine the other characteristics of the creature-to-be.

However, in relation to reproduction, humans are uncomfortable with family creation by close relatives. Reproduction by close relatives enhances the odds of life-threatening characteristics emerging in offspring. But what is it that attracts more distant people to other people? How are our drives to reproduce regulated? Humans still don't know why some persons find certain characteristics attractive and others unattractive, but much of this seems to be tied in with the need to not lose genetic characteristics within the larger gene pool. This tendency within nature to try to preserve a great variety of genetic characteristics may be at risk as humans are able to predetermine genetic characteristics prior to the birth of a baby. Effectively handling this ability to bypass nature's mechanisms for preservation of variation in the gene pool will be one of the important tests of whether humanity will be able to survive and thrive in the centuries to come.

Integumentary System

The skin, which is the basis of the integumentary system, protects all that lies underneath, provides us with our external appearance, and helps to regulate our temperature, preserving our very nature as warm-blooded creatures. It is also responsible for keeping fluids, minerals, proteins, and the many other necessary internal substances inside the body. Our blood cells circulate within us because the skin covers vascular beds. Skin also helps regulate our body temperature. It allows us to sweat—to lose substances that are present in overabundant supply. Evaporation of sweat from the skin's surface cools us in hot weather. "Goose bumps" protect us from heat loss through the skin in winter.

Skin characteristics, particularly around the face, have also signified identifying characteristics of the various human cultural and racial groups of our planet. It is unknown whether there is some sort of survival characteristic involved with this type of human-to-human recognition.

Following the additional round of practice with science questions in this chapter and a brief section on the sciences involved with the study of human behavior, such as sociology and psychology, there will be three sample tests. These sample tests, or model examinations, in Chapter Seven will reinforce the knowledge you have gained from earlier chapters. If you consider that some experts feel that each item on a multiple-choice test should take approximately one minute, you may want to time yourself. In language recall areas, such as vocabulary or spelling exercises, it would usually take less than a minute per item. At the other end of the time range would be reading comprehension items. To read a long paragraph and answer 30 reading comprehension items, you would want to allow 75 minutes.

Practice with Science Questions

Directions: Review the material on cells, tissues, organs, and body systems and then answer the following questions.

1. The process by which substances in solution pass from an area of higher concentration to an area of lower concentration is known as

   (A) diffusion.
   (B) osmosis.
   (C) oncotic pressure.
   (D) hydrostatic pressure.

2. Water is drawn from an area of low colloidal pressure to an area of higher colloidal pressure by a process known as

   (A) diffusion.
   (B) osmosis.
   (C) oncotic pressure.
   (D) hydrostatic pressure.

3. Which of the following are involved with movement of substances as the bloodstream, interstitium, and cells function to perform delivery and exchange?

   (A) Diffusion.
   (B) Osmosis.
   (C) Hydrostatic pressure.
   (D) All the above.

4. Which of the following blood cells are directly involved with the clotting process?

   (A) White cells.
   (B) Red cells.
   (C) Platelets.
   (D) Stem cells.

5. Which of the following are functions that cells are able to perform?

   (A) Taking in nutrients and oxygen.
   (B) Excreting byproducts of metabolism.
   (C) Synthesizing complex things.
   (D) All the above.

6. From the following list, which set of structures is organized from smallest to largest?

   (A) Cells, organs, tissues, systems.
   (B) Cells, tissues, organs, systems.
   (C) Tissues, organs, systems, cells.
   (D) Systems, organs, tissues, cells.

7. The six types of tissue are

   (A) epithelial, connective, reproductive, blood, muscle, nerve.
   (B) sensory, motor, afferent, efferent, central, peripheral.
   (C) frontal, sigmoid, sphenoid, deltoid, ethmoid, caretenoid.
   (D) None of the above.

8. Which of the following are organ systems of the human body?

   (A) Central, peripheral.
   (B) Afferent, efferent.
   (C) Stomach, lungs.
   (D) Integumentary, cardiorespiratory.

9. Impulses move throughout the nervous system by means of

   (A) a small electric current.
   (B) transmitter substances.
   (C) lymphatic vessels.
   (D) None of the above.

10. Which of the following ranks tissues according to regeneration ability, beginning with those that grow most rapidly and easily and ending with those that do not regenerate well when damaged.

    (A) Epithelial, muscle, nervous.
    (B) Muscle, epithelial, nervous.
    (C) Nervous, epithelial, muscle.
    (D) Epithelial, nervous, muscle.

11. Which of the following sets of statements is false?

    (A) Sensory nerves carry impulses from the peripheral areas of the body to the central nervous system. They are known as afferent nerves.
    (B) Efferent or motor nerves carry impulses toward the periphery.
    (C) Activation of the parasympathetic nervous system results in the fight-or-flight response.
    (D) Autonomic impulses are largely involuntary; somatic are voluntary.

12. Which is a correct analogy?

    (A) anterior pituitary : TSH :: posterior pituitary : ACTH.
    (B) anterior pituitary : ACTH :: posterior pituitary : ADH.
    (C) adrenal cortex : cortisone :: adrenal medulla : ADH.
    (D) adrenal cortex : adrenaline :: adrenal medulla : cortisone.

13. Which of the following statements is characteristic of sympathetic nervous system responses?

    (A) The air passages dilate, and the heart speeds up.
    (B) The body is ready for a nap.
    (C) The person will bleed more freely, and digestion will speed up.
    (D) The ability to see at closer range improves, and hearing is less acute.

14. Which of the following are not nutrient substances?

    (A) Fats.
    (B) Proteins.
    (C) Solvents.
    (D) Carbohydrates.

15. What is the function of bile?

    (A) Carbohydrate digestion.
    (B) Fat digestion.
    (C) Protein digestion.
    (D) Hormone digestion.

16. The pyloric sphincter lies between the

    (A) right atrium and right ventricle.
    (B) kidneys and bladder.
    (C) pancreas and small intestine.
    (D) stomach and duodenum/small intestine.

17. The stomach operates to digest food by which of the following processes?

    (A) Osmosis and diffusion.
    (B) Grinding (mechanical) and enzymatic/acidic (chemical).
    (C) Absorption and diffusion/permeability.
    (D) Excretion and dissolution.

18. In relation to final products into which major food groups are converted in order to pass into the bloodstream, which is a true statement?

    (A) Carbohydrates become simple sugars, such as glucose and sucrose.
    (B) Fats become fatty acids and glycerol.
    (C) Proteins become amino acids.
    (D) All of the statements are true.

19. Trace blood as it passes from the lungs to the body and back.

    (A) Lungs, left atrium, left ventricle, aorta (to the body), right atrium, right ventricle, and back to the lungs.
    (B) Lungs, right atrium, right ventricle, to the body, left atrium, left ventricle, and back to the lungs.
    (C) Lungs, right coronary artery, ventricles, atria, and back to the lungs.
    (D) Lungs, arteries, capillaries, and veins.

20. What is the respiratory membrane across which oxygen and carbon dioxide diffuse?

    (A) Diaphragm.
    (B) Oxygen-exchange membrane.
    (C) Alveolar-capillary.
    (D) Epithelial membrane.

21. What is the name given to the collecting tubules of the kidney?

    (A) Renal arteries.
    (B) Ureters.
    (C) Glomeruli.
    (D) Renal veins.

22. Which of the following are routinely excreted by the kidneys?

    (A) Proteins.
    (B) Simple sugars.
    (C) Electrolytes.
    (D) Red blood cells.

23. Genes, chromosomes, and sperm or egg cells are all involved in reproduction.
    Of these, which are the smallest?

    (A) Genes.
    (B) Chromosomes.
    (C) Sperm.
    (D) Egg.

24. The XY chromosome is characteristic of which of the following?

    (A) Genetic abnormality.
    (B) Males.
    (C) Females.
    (D) Blue eyes.

25. Which of the following are functions of the skin?

    (A) Protection.
    (B) Internal temperature control.
    (C) Conservation of internal substances.
    (D) All the above.

26. Approximately how many base pairs does the human genome contain?

    (A) Two thousand
    (B) Two million
    (C) Three billion
    (D) Three trillion

27. Human Genome Project (HGP) identified approximately how many genes in
    the human genome?

    (A) 2,000–3,000
    (B) 5,000–10,000
    (C) 10,000–20,000
    (D) 20,000–25,000

28. Which of the following does genetic mapping relate to?

    (A) Establishes sites of the gene on a chromosome.
    (B) Establishes four stages in gene variation.
    (C) Establishes the stages during cell division.
    (D) Illustrates various species in different regions.

Answers:

1. **(A)** Diffusion

2. **(B)** Osmosis

3. **(D)** Diffusion, osmosis, and hydrostatic pressure are all involved with delivery and exchange.

4. **(C)** Platelets are involved with clotting.

5. **(D)** Cells perform the following functions: taking in nutrients, taking in oxygen, excreting byproducts of metabolism, synthesizing complex things and releasing energy, regulating the internal environment (pH and temperature), moving or allowing internal movement, and reproducing.

6. **(B)** Cells are the smallest structures, followed by tissues and organs. Systems are the largest structures.

7. **(A)** Tissues can be epithelial, connective, reproductive, blood, muscle, or nerve.

8. **(D)** The organ systems are neuroendocrine, musculoskeletal, gastrointestinal, cardiorespiratory, renal/urinary, reproductive, and integumentary.

9. **(B)** Impulses move through the nervous system via transmitter substances.

10. **(A)** Epithelial tissue regenerates most rapidly, followed by muscle tissue and then nervous tissue, which can be nonregenerative in some areas.

11. **(C)** Activation of the sympathetic nervous system is associated with fight-or-flight.

12. **(B)** ACTH is secreted by the anterior pituitary and ADH by the posterior.

13. **(A)** The air passages dilate and the heart speeds up. This reaction is typical of the adrenaline response to perceived threat. The other responses are more characteristic of reactions produced by the parasympathetic system's activities.

14. **(C)** Solvents are not nutrients.

15. **(B)** Bile assists with fat digestion.

16. **(D)** The pyloric sphincter can be found between the stomach and the duodenum, or the stomach and the small intestine.

17. **(B)** The stomach uses mechanical (grinding of food into a paste) and chemical (action of acid and of enzymes) processes.

18. **(D)** Carbohydrates become simple sugars, such as glucose and sucrose. Fats become fatty acids and glycerol. Proteins become amino acids.

19. **(A)** From the lungs, blood will pass through the left side of the heart as it travels to the body.

20. **(C)** Oxygen and carbon dioxide diffuse across the alveolar-capillary membrane.

21. **(C)** Glomeruli

22. **(C)** Proteins, simple sugars, and red blood cells should be absent from urine.

23. **(A)** Genes are smaller (thousands per cell) than chromosomes, which are arrangements of genes (46 chromosomes in human cells). Sperm and egg cells are the largest of all.

24. **(B)** XY is male. XX is female.

25. **(D)** The skin protects, conserves, and assists with temperature control.

26. **(C)** There are three billion base pairs of the human genome.

27. **(D)** There are approximately 20,000–25,000 genes in the human genome.

28. **(A)** Genetic mapping establishes sites of the gene on a chromosome.

Systems Theory, Sociology, and Psychology

Now that you have had a chance to review the fundamental science concepts essential to nursing, a brief look at the behavioral sciences will help you put human activity into perspective. In animals and humans alike, we can visualize overall adjustment ability. Each organism must get along in its own environment. This ability to get along, responding appropriately to external and internal needs for change, is called adaptation. Coping is a related concept but refers to a shorter-term ability to respond to a need for change.

The living system can be thought of as something with boundaries that receives input and releases output back into the environment around it. In order to cope effectively, the organism receives signals (feedback) to alert the organism or a segment of the organism to a need for altering something. By using input, output, and feedback, organisms can adapt to and survive in the environment around them. These mechanisms encompass systems theory and have been useful in helping us understand and create behaviors for some of our more advanced computer systems. But more importantly, this theory allows us to break down and simplify human behaviors even though they are complex.

Sociology is the study of humans in groups. Nurses at the dawn of the twenty-first century will need to understand sociology because much of what they will do will involve influencing groups of people to remain healthier or to return to a state of personal high-level functioning. They will use such techniques as simple teaching and information linkage, but they will also need to understand why some groups are reluctant to alter behaviors to preserve their health. Sociologists know that humans tend to behave as those around them do. When people choose not to follow certain health-associated patterns, there is usually a set of identifiable reasons. The study of sociology allows for prediction and some degree of precision in encouraging groups to practice more healthful behaviors.

For example, the nurse who is working in a clinic or emergency room may note the prevalence of risk-taking behavior among teens. Combining a knowledge of sociology, growth and development, and teaching-learning principles, the nurse may be able to formulate a plan to bring a certain message into high schools in order to alter some of the students' riskiest behaviors. Because the public tends to perceive nurses as trustworthy, these teaching efforts may be at least partially successful.

One area of sociological knowledge that is especially important for nurses in the United States is that of cultural diversity. Nurses care for people who come from many countries and many cultures. Nurses must sometimes perform interventions that may seem a bit personal. It is important to know cultural differences. For example, knowing basic terms used by non-English speakers is often helpful in health care situations. It can be important to know how to obtain the services of a clinic or hospital interpreter. It can make a difference when one must explain or must institute care measures. Knowing in which cultures touch is considered an intrusion, or knowing the preferred personal space within differing cultures can prevent undue discomfort for patients and family members. Even eye contact or the asking of personal questions may have unintended connotations, depending on cultural background.

In contrast to sociology and its study of group behavior, psychology involves the study of individual human behavior. It involves identification of behaviors that are functional, or useful, as opposed to those that are dysfunctional. Nurses often encounter people under stress. People who seek health services often do so because they are ill or suspect that they may be ill. Not only is there stress related to possible illness and its effects, but there is also stress involved with entering the health care system, with its strange rituals, delays, and possibly uncomfortable environment or procedures. Nurses who understand this stress can help alleviate it.

In addition, nurses who understand the principles of psychology can recognize common coping mechanisms in themselves and others. Nurses are often able to recognize descent into some form of dysfunctional behavior, such as chemical abuse or one of the neuroses or psychoses. As the largest health care group in the country, nurses, individually, are in a position to interact with hundreds, or even thousands, of individuals each year. The possibility of assisting in meaningful ways depends on the sound integration of biological and behavioral sciences as a foundation for nursing practice.

Ethics

Before concluding our work with the sciences, it will be appropriate to consider the study of ethics. Although formal testing in ethics is often reserved for later study after entry into a nursing program, it is necessary to mention this aspect of preparation as early as possible in the career pathway of those choosing nursing as a life work.

Much has been said about the role of the sciences in a person's preparation for the nursing entrance examination and pursuit of a career in the helping professions. The study of ethics has emerged in recent times as a needed grounding for those who are engaged in the scientific or helping professions. There is a concern that the study of science and scientific principles in isolation does not prepare individuals for making decisions involving human life and death or the quality of existence. There has long been a concern that the scientist who has little contact with the world of political or ethical decision making may not consider the impact of his or her work on the real world outside the laboratory. There is a concern that the discoveries of modern science have an equal potential for doing great harm and great good in the world.

Nursing is very much a point-of-contact profession. The nurse is delivering a direct service, and the best of the institutions with which the nurse aligns ask the nurse, on a regular basis, to formulate and to modify plans for the care of the individual with direct input from the individual. Nursing is an altruistic profession, placing the good of the individual who is served above the immediate benefits of the nurse who provides the service. This quality of altruism is recognized, ultimately, by the public that permits nursing to have a certain level of autonomy within realistic societal boundaries. This sense of altruism dates from the beginnings of the profession. It permeates nursing and sets the profession apart in the modern world.

Ethical principles guide action. The three recognized categories of principles in ethical study are beneficence, justice, and respect for autonomy. Many of the consent forms that a patient signs to agree to treatments or procedures rest on principles of beneficence, justice, and autonomy. When a health care person explains things to patients and families, risks and benefits are often discussed. This is necessary to ensure that those who place their well-being in the hands of others are fully informed so that wise and informed choices might be made by those who will be most affected by the decisions made.

Beneficence is the first of the ethical principles used by health care personnel. It is the attempt to ensure that good is done. A part of beneficence is nonmaleficence, the attempt to, above all, do no harm. The last phrase is contained in the physician credo, "Primum non nocere," and is a cornerstone for health care personnel in all countries.

The second ethical principle, that of justice, involves treating others with fairness. The wise nurse's routine daily habit of examining his or her own motives helps the nurse avoid treating people with anything less than fairness. Modern hospitals definitely have written policies that spell out fairness and often have ethics councils to which nurses may refer questionable cases or practices. Being truthful and maintaining confidentiality are aspects of treating patients and families with an eye to maintaining the principle of justice.

Finally, the third ethical principle of respect for autonomy means honoring the rights of human beings to make decisions for themselves. This self-decision-making is curtailed by the proviso "as long as no needless harm is done to others." One could see this principle in action by observing the history of massive levels of smoking cessation in the United States in the final two decades of the twentieth century. Until the latter part of the century, people believed that those who smoked cigarettes were only harming themselves. Therefore, society ignored those individuals who chose to smoke because it was their autonomous decision to engage in an unhealthy practice. Since it was believed that they did no harm to others, the practice was permitted. After scientific evidence tilted in the direction of grave harm from inhaling smoke exhaled by the smoker (second-hand smoke), society took another look. What had seemed harmless to the general population was probably not. A series of changes in social practice and in the law resulted in such practical outcomes as no smoking in confined spaces, such as airplanes, hospitals, and restaurants. One could still respect the autonomy of the smoker by allowing smoking outside of buildings, but society recognized that indoor smoking violated others' rights to fresh air and to not be harmed by another's choices.

The three ethical principles of beneficence, justice, and respect for autonomy continue to be applied in almost all aspects of human endeavor. However, they are not always easily applied in each individual case. Therefore, there is a specialized body of study and interpretation. Interpreting principles of ethics and applying them to the lives of individuals in everyday situations of health and illness is the work of bioethicists. Most larger hospitals and health care corporations have groups of ethicists who meet on a regular basis to formulate guidelines to be used in difficult situations.

Nurses are aware that current bioethical issues center around the beginning of life and the end of life. Such issues as abortion, contraception, in vitro fertilization, surrogate mothering, and genetic research have come to the fore in the modern world as a result of scientific advances. Examples of ethical issues centering around the end of life are the determination of when life ends, including definitions of death; active euthanasia, the causing of death through the use of outside intervention; and care of persons with diseases brought about through avoidable behaviors. Should insurance premiums be higher for those who smoke cigarettes? What about those who eat a diet that contains foods known to be associated with early onset of heart disease? Will insurance premiums be lower one day for those who ride bikes to work? For those who live in the countryside? All of these questions might one day come under the scope of ethical decision making.

Sometimes it seems that the pace of change as a result of new scientific and technical advances threatens to overwhelm the abilities of modern ethical institutions to develop guidelines. In addition to beginning-of-life and end-of-life concerns, there are issues involving access to health care. That is, will health care be available for all people at equal levels of effectiveness, or will society permit inequities in accessing services or in the delivery of services? In other words, will there be tiers of health care, some for rich and some for poor? Insurance and insurability are also hot topics in the United States at the dawn of the twenty-first century. There are moves afoot to ration health care or to curtail the extent of services that will be provided for those who have a small chance of survival.

Finally, ethical issues of concern to nurses include the environment and management of exposure to hazards. One could even stretch current ethical concerns to include the newer nursing field of study, that of disaster management. In a time of mass casualties, how does the nurse performing triage sort out who will be treated first and who will not? How does the nurse direct services? Triage, or the sorting of victims into three groups based on survivability and pressing need for health care attention, is based on the ethical principle of utilitarianism: the greatest good for the greatest number. How does the nurse decide when the assignment of health care services may safely return to normal, the treating of all in need, and away from rigid triage principles? All of this is part of modern health teaching for the nurse.

Leah Curtin has devised three levels of decision making for the nurse or others involved in the provision of health care services. The most desirable level is deliberative decision making. With deliberative decision making, the provider of services is able to formulate a carefully thought-out plan, checking with all stakeholders to see that the plan is acceptable. In formulating the plan, there is no pressing time limit. Background works are read, experts are consulted, the family and patient are fully consulted, and committees of learned persons have time to deliberate. Much of the time, Curtin's intermediate level is called for in nursing. The nurse relies on the background work of others who have formulated plans for most situations likely to arise. The nurse may be able to access persons who have specialized training in such situations. But, moderately fast action must occur. The immediate level of decision making, the third and most rapid, occurs when there is little time for overt, paced thought. In the end, the nurse will make a quick and hopefully accurate decision, say, as the side-of-the-road accident has just occurred or victims of the explosion or fire are brought to his or her facility for immediate treatment. Training and modern communications, allowing access to others trained in rapid response, will help to support nurses' decisions in such emergency situations. But, with all levels of decision making, ethical dilemmas may occur, and ethical themes are apparent. The nurse hopes to do no harm, but certainly risk will increase when situations call for immediate action.

Benner characterizes the progress of a nurse from novice to expert through five levels of development. The levels are novice, advanced beginner, competent, proficient, and expert provider of care. Student nurses are exposed to more independent decision making as they approach the level of novice nurse. Following graduation and the passing of a specialized nursing examination, nurses will achieve novice status within several months to a year. This situation may not make ethical decision making easy in all cases, but there will always be guidelines and the opportunity for referral to others who are experienced and specifically trained to assist in this challenging work. There are even specialized nurses known as nurse ethicists who work within major hospitals in the United States. Nurses, as the around-the-clock care givers in hospitals or the long-term contacts who may know patients best when they are outside hospitals, are in a pivotal position to discover situations in which ethics expertise may be required.

Answer Sheet
SAMPLE TEST

Science

1 Ⓐ Ⓑ Ⓒ Ⓓ   6 Ⓐ Ⓑ Ⓒ Ⓓ   11 Ⓐ Ⓑ Ⓒ Ⓓ
2 Ⓐ Ⓑ Ⓒ Ⓓ   7 Ⓐ Ⓑ Ⓒ Ⓓ   12 Ⓐ Ⓑ Ⓒ Ⓓ
3 Ⓐ Ⓑ Ⓒ Ⓓ   8 Ⓐ Ⓑ Ⓒ Ⓓ   13 Ⓐ Ⓑ Ⓒ Ⓓ
4 Ⓐ Ⓑ Ⓒ Ⓓ   9 Ⓐ Ⓑ Ⓒ Ⓓ   14 Ⓐ Ⓑ Ⓒ Ⓓ
5 Ⓐ Ⓑ Ⓒ Ⓓ   10 Ⓐ Ⓑ Ⓒ Ⓓ   15 Ⓐ Ⓑ Ⓒ Ⓓ

Science Sample Test

Directions: Read the following paragraphs and answer the questions. This first section is a timed test. At the end of one minute of reading, mark the spot where you stopped when time was called and then continue on for seven more minutes. You should be able to complete the whole passage well within the eight-minute time limit. The interpretation of the one-minute test score is given at the end of this sample test. Set up your time-keeping system and begin.

The Sociologic Concept of Stress

Stress is considered to be a problem for human beings in the twenty-first century. There is a feeling in the Western world that the numbers and types of stressful events (termed stressors) are increasing as technology begins to permeate almost all facets of life and as what is considered relaxation time begins to blend with work time. Stress is to be distinguised from certain related terms. While stress is a prevailing condition, the precipitating event causing the condition is a stressor. As an example, getting a very large bill from a company for things you didn't buy would be a stressor. It would create the condition of stress, or the stress reaction. It would set up a condition in which the individual feels forced to act in order to relieve feelings of discomfort. Acting to relieve stress is termed coping. Coping may involve both acting to relieve or get rid of the stressor or, in humans, calming the associated feelings of discomfort. Often, coping involves both types of stress-reduction at the same time: getting rid of stressors and handling associated emotions.

The nineteenth-century pioneers in stress research include Claude Bernard, who did early research on the biologic need for maintenance of stability in the internal environment, and Walter B. Cannon, who coined such terms as "homeostasis" and "fight or flight." These two researchers used animals, primarily, for their research, as did Hans Selye, an early twentieth-century pioneer in stress research. Hans Selye described a general response to stressors known as the General Adaptation Syndrome. He described internal changes in physical reaction, discriminating, for the first time, between stressor and stress. He noted a variety of consistent internal responses to stress-producing stimuli. Some of the internal changes precipitated during the stress response are alike for both animals and humans. These are a heightened sense of alertness, dilated pupils to enhance distance vision, faster respiratory rate and opening out of the respiratory passages, higher blood pressure, shunting of blood supply to brain and skeletal muscles so that flight may be accomplished or a fight can be won, and setting up mechanisms so that blood will clot quickly in case of injury. All this persists during the stress response but will slowly abate after the need passes.

Lazarus and Folkman, long after Freud's work examining the human psyche, and following the early stress work with lab animals, forged a coherent theory of how the human being perceived, interpreted, and reacted in situations of stress. One salient point involved an intermediate step between the human individual's initial noting of a potentially threatening situation (arousal) and the actual stress reaction. This intermediate step was called appraisal and was a determination of whether a threat existed and whether the person could do anything about it.

Three major types of stress events have been identified. One is the cataclysmic event, first intensively studied and described by Lindemann after the Coconut Grove fire in the 1940s. The second and third types of stress conditions are life change events and daily hassles. Life change events, important major life alterations, were described and measured by Holmes and Rahe (1976), and the more minor but annoying events known as daily hassles were described by Lazarus and Folkman (1989).

It is logical to believe that mankind will continue to deal with all of these types of stressors. Humanity is constructed to survive in the presence of even the heaviest of stress burdens and the most intensive quantities of individual daily stressors. One day, historians and archeologists of the future will marvel at either the tremendous ability of twenty-first-century humans to live in the midst of powerful and unrelenting stress or will be envious of what could be considered, by future historians, to be a remarkably placid period for mankind.

1. Which of the following defines the word *stressor*?

   (A) a stimulus
   (B) something causing the stress reaction
   (C) the stress reaction
   (D) fight or flight

2. What is thought to be the relationship between modern living and stress?

   (A) As modern life, with its high technology, goes on, stressful events tend to increase in individuals' lives.
   (B) Modern living, with all its conveniences, means diminished stress levels for humanity.
   (C) There is no relationship between stress and modern life. Nothing's been proven.
   (D) Coping is situation-based.

3. Which stress researchers performed the majority of their experiments exclusively on animals?

   (A) Cannon, Selye
   (B) Lazarus, Folkman
   (C) Peplau, Nightingale
   (D) Holmes, Rahe

4. Who concluded that, in humans, the intermediate step of appraisal precedes taking action and follows alerting?

(A) Cannon
(B) Bernard
(C) Selye
(D) Lazarus

5. Which internal changes happen during the stress response?

(A) The throat closes up in fear, and the person has trouble concentrating.
(B) The person runs away, if possible, or prepares to fight.
(C) Heart beat becomes faster, and air passages dilate to let in more air.
(D) The person sweats heavily and will become tired easily if the response continues.

6. What are the most likely choices for occurrences following appraisal?

(A) stress response, panic, alarm
(B) stopping current activity and going to investigate
(C) continued appraisal, hyperventilation
(D) relaxation (no threat), stress response, or continued appraisal

Stop at this point to ensure that you were able to read the material on stress and were able to answer the questions within the total time of eight minutes. If you reached line 45 within the first minute, you are a fast reader; if you reached line 33, you are a moderate reader; if you did not reach line 33, you are a slow reader and will need to practice reading more often. Answers to the stress section are provided at the end.

Public Health Concepts

Some mosquitoes carry the virus that causes encephalitis, a deadly swelling of the brain for which there is no effective preventive vaccine or treatment. The disease may cause death in up to 30 percent of those infected. It is prevalent in areas of the country in which mosquitoes breed easily and in which people tend to live outdoors during much of the year.

7. In general, one would expect to notice highest rates of occurrence of encephalitis in

   (A) Alaska.
   (B) Florida.
   (C) New Mexico.
   (D) Kansas.

8. If one were living or visiting in a part of the country in which there was an encephalitis outbreak, which of the following measures might be most effective and practical at preventing the disease?

   (A) Stay indoors in the evening when most mosquitoes are active.
   (B) Make sure that you are immunized with an annual vaccination.
   (C) Wear heavier clothing.
   (D) Do not go swimming.

First Aid/CPR

Most states have "Good Samaritan" laws, which allow persons to stop at the scene of an accident and to render assistance without fear of legal reprisal. Individuals may assist as would a person using ordinary good judgment and acting in good faith. For example, the helpful person might decide to apply pressure to a profusely bleeding arm wound to stop the bleeding. This would constitute using ordinary good judgment. However, it would be questionable if the lay person assisting at the scene decided to move a person lying at the side of the road, in no immediate danger, but who appeared to have recently fallen off a motorcycle. Moving such a person might lead to an increase in possible spinal area injuries.

9. In the context of this paragraph, what would be the meaning of the word *reprisal*?

   (A) a prison sentence
   (B) a reprimand
   (C) having negative action brought to bear as a consequence of one's behavior
   (D) notoriety, as in having one's name appear in published documents open to public scrutiny

10. In the context of this paragraph, what is the meaning of the term *lay*?

    (A) nonprofessional
    (B) resting
    (C) religious
    (D) nonreligious

11. Which of the following actions would be safe in the case of a car wreck in which gasoline fumes are apparent, as well as a pool of gasoline surrounding the car? The one unconscious victim seems to be lying under the car but is not pinned underneath.

    (A) Do not move the person lest you injure the spine. Try to find water to dilute any gasoline in the area.
    (B) With other people who have arrived on the scene, move the person away from the car.
    (C) Tell the person that help is on the way, but take no other action. Make sure someone has called 911.
    (D) Keep the crowds back from the scene of the accident.

Anatomy and Physiology

In science, one begins to notice a pattern to the shape and location of internal organs, whether the creature under consideration is human or another variety of animal-kingdom inhabitant. For example, all animal-kingdom species possess a food tube. Whether one is dealing with a lowly worm or a sea-dwelling eel, the food tube and its appendages are used to scoop in food from the external environment and to rid the body of unnecessary elements.

12. Which of the following statements explains the presence, at a microscopic level, of the corrugated or wrinkled appearance of the interior of the intestines (rather than their being more like a smooth tube)?

    (A) They must grind food into small particles.
    (B) This feature protects the intestinal surface against damage from acidic foods.
    (C) This is a gravity-assist device.
    (D) A larger surface area is exposed to nutrients which will be absorbed into the bloodstream.

13. Which of the following statements is logical with respect to the placement of the heart within the chest cavity rather than within the abdomen?

    (A) The heart needs to be near the brain to ensure a steady supply of nutrients to the brain.
    (B) The heart needs to be protected from trauma.
    (C) The heart and lungs must work in synchrony and, therefore, must be located near each other.
    (D) The heart developed when sea creatures began to dwell on land.

14. Which of the following *best* explains why there are small one-way valves in human leg veins, which carry blood back to the heart, but not in the leg veins of frogs?

    (A) Frogs are primitive. Humans are not.
    (B) Even after death or separation of a frog's legs from its body, an electric current will continue to make the leg jump.
    (C) This is a gravity-assist device.
    (D) Lighter-skinned creatures have more fragile veins.

15. In comparison with other members of the animal kingdom, which is the best explanation for the human tendency to develop low back pain more often?

    (A) Humans have an upright gait (walk erect).
    (B) Humans don't possess a tail.
    (C) The weight of the human brain is greater than that of other members of the animal kingdom.
    (D) Humans have poor posture.

Science Sample Test Answer Key

1. **(B)** This is simple recall from early in the reading on stress.

2. **(A)** Readings show stressful events are a more modern concern.

3. **(A)** Cannon and Selye were earliest and worked primarily with laboratory animals. Later researchers used human participants with their wider range of responses to stressors.

4. **(D)** Lazarus, the more recent of the listed researchers, was the one who worked with humans rather than animals.

5. **(C)** This is an internal, immediate, and generalized response to a stressor.

6. **(D)** Following arousal, living beings appraise a threat, no threat, or will continue to gather information.

7. **(B)** Encephalitis would be more prevalent in Florida, since people live outdoors longer and mosquitoes breed more easily due to warm climate and relatively high moisture levels.

8. **(A)** Since the information given on encephalitis states there is no effective vaccine, B would be incorrect. D has little to do with this disease's transmission. Of the remaining choices, A makes more sense.

9. **(C)** Any answer could be a reprisal, but the one most closely associated with Good Samaritan laws is the generic negative action.

10. **(A)** Since the paragraph did not deal with religious faith, the most likely choice would be "nonprofessional."

11. **(B)** Although it is wiser not to move accident victims, this special circumstance would cause rescuers to weigh what course of action is less dangerous. Very careful bracing of the head, neck, and back, using many rescuers operating in synchronous fashion, should allow for a safe move.

12. **(D)** The reader would note the term "microscopic level" and choose an answer that has to do with very small units of food—the molecular level.

13. **(B)** The rib cage protects this absolutely vital organ. Abdominal organs can withstand trauma long enough for recovery to occur and the person can survive for days with a dysfunctional intestinal system, but the heart must beat relatively regularly during each minute over the course of a lifetime.

14. **(C)** Humans walk upright and need this bit of extra assistance with returning blood from the legs up to the heart.

15. **(A)** While the lumbar area of the spinal column has the thickest and strongest bones, a lifetime of walking upright and of using the upper body to push and pull will place great tension in the lower back area.

Answer Sheet
NUMERICAL ABILITY TEST

Numerical Ability

1 Ⓐ Ⓑ Ⓒ Ⓓ	18 Ⓐ Ⓑ Ⓒ Ⓓ	35 Ⓐ Ⓑ Ⓒ Ⓓ
2 Ⓐ Ⓑ Ⓒ Ⓓ	19 Ⓐ Ⓑ Ⓒ Ⓓ	36 Ⓐ Ⓑ Ⓒ Ⓓ
3 Ⓐ Ⓑ Ⓒ Ⓓ	20 Ⓐ Ⓑ Ⓒ Ⓓ	37 Ⓐ Ⓑ Ⓒ Ⓓ
4 Ⓐ Ⓑ Ⓒ Ⓓ	21 Ⓐ Ⓑ Ⓒ Ⓓ	38 Ⓐ Ⓑ Ⓒ Ⓓ
5 Ⓐ Ⓑ Ⓒ Ⓓ	22 Ⓐ Ⓑ Ⓒ Ⓓ	39 Ⓐ Ⓑ Ⓒ Ⓓ
6 Ⓐ Ⓑ Ⓒ Ⓓ	23 Ⓐ Ⓑ Ⓒ Ⓓ	40 Ⓐ Ⓑ Ⓒ Ⓓ
7 Ⓐ Ⓑ Ⓒ Ⓓ	24 Ⓐ Ⓑ Ⓒ Ⓓ	41 Ⓐ Ⓑ Ⓒ Ⓓ
8 Ⓐ Ⓑ Ⓒ Ⓓ	25 Ⓐ Ⓑ Ⓒ Ⓓ	42 Ⓐ Ⓑ Ⓒ Ⓓ
9 Ⓐ Ⓑ Ⓒ Ⓓ	26 Ⓐ Ⓑ Ⓒ Ⓓ	43 Ⓐ Ⓑ Ⓒ Ⓓ
10 Ⓐ Ⓑ Ⓒ Ⓓ	27 Ⓐ Ⓑ Ⓒ Ⓓ	44 Ⓐ Ⓑ Ⓒ Ⓓ
11 Ⓐ Ⓑ Ⓒ Ⓓ	28 Ⓐ Ⓑ Ⓒ Ⓓ	45 Ⓐ Ⓑ Ⓒ Ⓓ
12 Ⓐ Ⓑ Ⓒ Ⓓ	29 Ⓐ Ⓑ Ⓒ Ⓓ	46 Ⓐ Ⓑ Ⓒ Ⓓ
13 Ⓐ Ⓑ Ⓒ Ⓓ	30 Ⓐ Ⓑ Ⓒ Ⓓ	47 Ⓐ Ⓑ Ⓒ Ⓓ
14 Ⓐ Ⓑ Ⓒ Ⓓ	31 Ⓐ Ⓑ Ⓒ Ⓓ	48 Ⓐ Ⓑ Ⓒ Ⓓ
15 Ⓐ Ⓑ Ⓒ Ⓓ	32 Ⓐ Ⓑ Ⓒ Ⓓ	49 Ⓐ Ⓑ Ⓒ Ⓓ
16 Ⓐ Ⓑ Ⓒ Ⓓ	33 Ⓐ Ⓑ Ⓒ Ⓓ	50 Ⓐ Ⓑ Ⓒ Ⓓ
17 Ⓐ Ⓑ Ⓒ Ⓓ	34 Ⓐ Ⓑ Ⓒ Ⓓ	

Model Examinations

CHAPTER 7

Numerical Ability Test

50 Test Items: TIME: 50 MINUTES

Directions: For each question, select the letter (A, B, C, or D) that corresponds to your answer. Mark your answer on the Numerical Ability Answer Sheet on page 253.

1. Mary is planning a pizza party for her son. The manager of the local pizza restaurant says one of his pizzas contains 14 slices. Mary is planning on inviting 15 of her son's friends to the party. How many large pizzas will Mary need to order if she figures each child attending the party will eat four pieces?

   (A) 4
   (B) 10
   (C) 7
   (D) 5

2. A woman is diagnosed as having a bacterial infection and is given a prescription for an antibiotic. The prescription instructs the woman to take 3 tablets daily for 18 days. The pharmacist tells the woman each antibiotic tablet costs $2.58. What will the woman pay for the prescription of antibiotics?

   (A) $46.44
   (B) $139.32
   (C) $54.00
   (D) $156.74

3. Select the response in which the fractions $\frac{15}{45}$, $\frac{18}{75}$, and $\frac{45}{60}$ are written from least to greatest.

   (A) $\frac{15}{45}$ $\frac{18}{75}$ $\frac{45}{60}$

   (B) $\frac{18}{75}$ $\frac{15}{45}$ $\frac{45}{60}$

   (C) $\frac{45}{60}$ $\frac{18}{75}$ $\frac{15}{45}$

   (D) $\frac{15}{45}$ $\frac{45}{60}$ $\frac{18}{75}$

4. Jackson is considering buying an insurance policy, but he cannot afford more than $500.00 a year in annual premiums. He is considering a $15,000 policy with an annual premium of $35 per $1,000. Can Jackson afford the policy?

   (A) No, the annual premium is $25 more than Jackson can afford.
   (B) No, the annual premium is $525 more than Jackson can afford.
   (C) Yes, the annual premium is exactly $500 a year.
   (D) Yes, Jackson could afford a policy valued at $18,500.

5. Lacy owns 800 shares of Congo Gold Mines Limited stock. The stock pays a dividend of $8.50 per share semiannually. How much will Lacy receive in dividends in one year?

   (A) $6,800
   (B) $13,600
   (C) $68
   (D) $136

6. A motorist drove at a speed of 55 miles per hour for five hours before stopping for a rest. After resting, the motorist drove at a speed of 65 miles per hour for six additional hours. What was the average miles per hour driven by the motorist?

   (A) 59.75 mph
   (B) 60 mph
   (C) 66.5 mph
   (D) 60.5 mph

7. $(4 \times 13) + (15 \times 8) =$

   (A) 399
   (B) 172
   (C) 40
   (D) 158

8. A hospital is looking into how nurses spend their time. Nurses are asked to keep track of time spent in four areas: (1) direct patient care, (2) preparing and administering medications, (3) assisting other health care professionals, and (4) nonpatient care activities. Results demonstrate that nurses spend three fifths of their time performing direct patient care, one eighth of their time preparing and administering medications, and one sixth of their time assisting other health care professionals. What percentage of the nurses' time was spent performing nonpatient care activities?

   (A) 20%
   (B) 12%
   (C) 19%
   (D) 11%

9. A circle has a circumference of 8 inches. The radius of the circle is

   (A) 1.25 inches.
   (B) 2.5 inches.
   (C) 25.12 inches.
   (D) .3925 inches.

10. What is the value of $17.3 + 5.75 - 16.02$?

    (A) 7.0
    (B) 7.03
    (C) 39.1
    (D) 6.82

11. A nurse's aide makes $5.58 an hour working the 7 A.M.–3 P.M. shift. She makes $6.00 an hour working the 3 P.M.–11 P.M. shift. What amount does she earn based on the following time card?

Monday	7:00 A.M.–11:20 A.M.
	12:20 P.M.–3:00 P.M.
Tuesday	3:00 P.M.–8:00 P.M.
	8:30 P.M.–11:00 P.M.
Wednesday	7:00 A.M.–11:00 P.M.

   (A) $176.70
   (B) $225.43
   (C) $170.19
   (D) $183.00

12. The normal dosage for a medication is 20 mg/kg/day. The patient weighs 50 kg. How much medication should the patient receive? Solve for x.

    (A) 1,000 mg
    (B) 200 mg
    (C) 1,500 mg
    (D) 900 mg

13. Philip has $3.00 to spend on marbles. One marble costs 37¢. How many marbles can Philip buy?

    (A) 10
    (B) 8
    (C) 5
    (D) 7

14. A man borrowed a sum of money with an interest rate of 8% annually for five years. At the end of five years, he had paid $500 in interest. What amount did the man borrow?

    (A) $2,000
    (B) $1,250
    (C) $3,125
    (D) $2,500

15. Bryan has $3,500 to pay for one semester of college. One third of his money will pay room and board, one fifth will pay for books and supplies, and one fourth will pay for tuition. Any money left will be spending money. How much will Bryan have for spending money?

    (A) $657.84
    (B) $758
    (C) $507.55
    (D) $800

16. What is the simple interest on $750 at 15% for 26 months?

    (A) $158.75
    (B) $4.33
    (C) $1,300
    (D) $244.13

17. Results of the biology exam indicated 89 students took the exam. The biology teacher told the class that one sixth of the class had failed the exam. Posted results of the exam indicated 15% of the class received above 90%. What is the difference between the number of students that failed the exam and the number of students who scored above 90% on the exam?

    (A) 80
    (B) 2
    (C) 15
    (D) 11

18. A graduate student is hired to double-check data collected by a researcher. There are 854 data sets to check. After learning the system, the graduate student can check 6 sets per hour. After 8 hours another graduate student is enlisted to speed the process of checking data sets. The second student can check 4.5 data sets per hour. How many total hours are needed to double-check all the data sets? Round to the nearest hour.

    (A) 81 hours
    (B) 85 hours
    (C) 77 hours
    (D) 90 hours

19. John and Penny have five children. Their youngest child is 5 years old and the oldest child is 30 years old. How old are the remaining children if the second child is 5 years older than the youngest child, the middle child is 15 years younger than the oldest child, and the fourth child is twice the age of the second?

    (A) 10, 15, and 20 years
    (B) 10, 12, and 24 years
    (C) 5, 10, and 20 years
    (D) 5, 15, and 30 years

20. A grocery store has a candy bin that sells various types of candy. Jaw Lockers sell for $2.50 a pound, Sour Cherries for $3.00 a half pound, Orange Blitzes for $1.50 a pound, and Goofy Gum for 75¢ a pound. What is the average cost per pound of the candy in the bin?

    (A) $2.69
    (B) $1.94
    (C) $3.00
    (D) $1.50

21. Virginia's monthly salary is $3,514. Taxes and social security deduct 34%. Her employer deducts $150 for repayment of a loan prior to issuing Virginia's check. How much does Virginia take home each month?

    (A) $2,169.24
    (B) $1,143.76
    (C) $1,245.76
    (D) $1,898.43

22. In April, 950 graduates of nursing programs took the licensure examination. Of these, 843 passed the examination. How many graduates were unsuccessful on the licensure examination?

    (A) 112
    (B) 68
    (C) 843
    (D) 107

23. Find the sum of $8 - 2 + (-10)$.

    (A) −4
    (B) 0
    (C) 20
    (D) 12

24. In $\triangle DEF$, the measure of $\angle D$ is four times the measure of $\angle F$. The measure of $\angle E$ is 2.5 times the measure of $\angle F$. What is the measure of $\angle F$?

    (A) 24°
    (B) 48°
    (C) 60°
    (D) 96°

25. Your monthly grocery bill increases from $157.65 to $298.60 when your son comes home from college. The percentage of increase is

    (A) 47.2%.
    (B) 141%.
    (C) 89.4%.
    (D) 57.7%.

26. A researcher is developing a new trail mix. The recipe contains 8 ounces of raisins, 6 ounces of pecans, 4 ounces of peanuts, and 5 ounces of dried fruit. How many more ounces of dried fruit must be added to make the trail mix 25% dried fruit in weight?

    (A) 3 ounces
    (B) 2.5 ounces
    (C) 4 ounces
    (D) 1 ounce

27. A patient is taking a medication ordered at 45 milliequivalents (meq) by mouth PO 4-times-per-day (qid) with juice. The medication is available as 30 meq/20 mL. How many mL of medication should be administered per dose?

    (A) 15 mL
    (B) 25 mL
    (C) 30 mL
    (D) 35 mL

28. A patient taking a blood pressure medication is not responding to therapy. The physician increases the blood pressure medication from 300 mg a day to 650 mg a day. What is the percentage of increase in blood pressure medication?

    (A) 117%
    (B) 100%
    (C) 46%
    (D) 216%

29. A hospital's central supply has 596 winter blankets on hand when an early snow storm strikes the area. Based on hospital census, one third of the blankets go to medical-surgical floors, one fifth go to critical care areas, and three sevenths of the blankets go to surgery. What fraction of the blankets will be left in central supply?

    (A) two thirds
    (B) one third
    (C) one twenty-fifth
    (D) one fourth

30. Bill bought 25 shares of Ski Copper Mountain stock at $5.85 a share. He sold the shares five years later at $46.50 a share. What is Bill's profit?

    (A) $1,162.50
    (B) $146.25
    (C) $1,016.25
    (D) $1,308.75

31. A telephone company needs to install a new antenna on the top of a building. The manager of the company does not know what height antenna to purchase because the original antenna records were lost. Installation records for the original antenna indicate that guide wires were placed 12 feet from the base of the antenna, and a total of 80 feet of wire was used for four supports. How tall an antenna does the manager need to order?

    (A) 8 feet
    (B) 12 feet
    (C) 16 feet
    (D) 32 feet

32. The student nurses' club is having their annual bake sale. They plan to sell 75 cupcakes for 50¢ apiece, 250 cookies for 25¢ apiece, 150 donuts for 60¢ apiece, and 150 donut holes for 15¢ apiece. If all the bake goods are sold, how much will the club make?

    (A) $212.50
    (B) $215.46
    (C) $208.40
    (D) $200.50

33. A manager of a shoe store bought a shipment of sandals for $20 a pair and sold the entire shipment for $148. The shoe store made $8.50 profit on each pair of sandals. How many pairs of sandals did the manager purchase?

    (A) 63
    (B) 7
    (C) 142
    (D) 15

34. $10 + 8 \times 15 + 10 \div 2 =$

    (A) 140
    (B) 170
    (C) 135
    (D) 157

35. A physician's order reads, "Give 1 gram of Penicillin before breakfast." The pharmacy is out of 1 gram tablets and sends tablets containing 125 mg of Penicillin per tablet. How many Penicillin tablets will the nurse administer before breakfast?

    (A) 12.5
    (B) 8
    (C) 10
    (D) 7

36. Select one-sixth percent written as a decimal.

    (A) 16%
    (B) 0.06%
    (C) 6%
    (D) 0.166%

37. The medication amount to be administered to a patient is 600 mg of Tylenol (acetaminophen). The order is written for grains (gr) × (10) PO every 3 hours. How many tablets of Tylenol will the nurse administer to the patient?

    (A) 1 tablet
    (B) ½ tablet
    (C) 2 tablets
    (D) 2.5 tablets

38. Solve for *x.* $15x + 6x - 3x + 18 = 26x$

    (A) 2.25
    (B) 9
    (C) 3
    (D) 1.38

39. A student makes the following grades on homework assignments: 78, 84, 56, 96, 78, 85, 85, 95, 0, 73. What is the student's average grade on the assignments?

    (A) 85
    (B) 73
    (C) 81
    (D) 96

40. $18 + 7(2 \times 6) - (6 + 3) =$

    (A) 93
    (B) 291
    (C) 192
    (D) 35

41. When five times a number is increased by 14 the result is 54. What is the number?

    (A) 13.6
    (B) 68
    (C) 8
    (D) 4

42. A newly married couple bought an old house in need of repair for $35,000. Over ten years they spent $20,000 refurbishing the house. After living in the house for many years, they sell the house for $65,000. How much profit did the couple make on the house?

    (A) $30,000
    (B) $45,000
    (C) $10,000
    (D) $15,000

43. A train is traveling at 86 miles per hour. How long will it take the train to reach a city 400 miles away?

    (A) 4 hours 42 minutes
    (B) 6 hours
    (C) 5 hours 4 minutes
    (D) 8 hours

44. What percent of 15 is 8?

    (A) 53%
    (B) 120%
    (C) 7%
    (D) 23%

45. Which of the following is the greatest common factor of 15, 48, and 63?

    (A) 5
    (B) 3
    (C) 4
    (D) 7

46. Central supply has the following items in stock:

    17 boxes of abdominal pads at $15 a box
    6 boxes of Band-aids at $7.50 a box
    43 boxes of alcohol pads at $4 a box
    150 boxes of tissues at $1.50 a box
    11 boxes of cloth tape at $8.40 a box

    Issued to the nursing units during one day were:

    10 boxes of abdominal pads
    5 boxes of bandaids
    18 boxes of alcohol pads
    10 boxes of tissues
    3 boxes of cloth tape

    What is the dollar amount of supplies issued to the nursing units?

    (A) $299.70
    (B) $354.32
    (C) $158.07
    (D) $340.85

47. Marcia works as a free-lance writer and sells her stories to the highest bidder. She recently wrote a story on the return of the buffalo herds to the Goodnight Ranch in Texas. Four magazines have made offers to purchase her story. Magazine A offered $458 minus 3% for editing, Magazine B offered $450 minus 2% for editing, Magazine C offered $480 minus 5% for editing, and Magazine D offered a flat $440 for the story. Which magazine will pay Marcia the greatest amount for her story?

(A) Magazine A
(B) Magazine B
(C) Magazine C
(D) Magazine D

48. What is the least common factor of 6, 10, and 15?

(A) 900
(B) 60
(C) 45
(D) 30

49. How many total inches are in 7 feet 4 inches and 4 feet 10 inches?

(A) 257 inches
(B) 130 inches
(C) 126 inches
(D) 146 inches

50. A box contains 3 colors of pencils. One fourth are black, three eighths are red, and the remaining 16 are yellow. How many pencils are in the box?

(A) 19
(B) 2
(C) 43
(D) 6

STOP

If there is still time remaining, you may review your answers.

NUMERICAL ABILITY TEST ANSWER KEY

1. **(D)** 1 child : 4 slices of pizza =
   16 children : x slices of pizza
                   $x = 64$ slices of pizza

   1 pizza : 14 slices = x pizza : 64 slices
                   $14x = 64$
                   $x = 4.57$ pizzas = 5 pizzas

2. **(B)** 1 tablet : $2.58 = 54 tablets : x
                   $x = \$139.32$

3. **(B)**

4. **(A)** Policy = $15,000
   Premium rate = $35/$1,000
   Annual premium = x

   $35 : $1,000 = x : $15,000
           $1,000x = 525,000$
               $x = \$525$

5. **(B)**

6. **(D)** 55 mph × 5 = 275 miles
   65 mph × 6 = 390 miles
   $$\left(\frac{275 + 390}{11}\right) = 60.45 = 60.5 \text{ mph}$$

7. **(B)**

8. **(D)**
   Least Common Multiple = 120

   $$\frac{3}{5} = \frac{72}{120} \quad \frac{1}{8} = \frac{15}{120} \quad \frac{1}{6} = \frac{20}{120}$$

   $$\frac{107}{120} = 89\%$$

   $100\% - 89\% = 11\%$

9. **(A)**
circumference = 8 inches
$\pi = 3.14$
diameter = unknown

$C = \pi d$
$8 = (3.14)(d)$
$2.5 = d$

radius = unknown
diameter = 2.5 inches

$r = \frac{1}{2}d$
$r = \left(\frac{1}{2}\right)(2.5)$
$r = 1.25$ inches

10. **(B)**

11. **(A)**

Monday:	7 A.M.–11:20 A.M. = 4.33 hours	
	12:20 P.M.–3 P.M. = 2.67 hours	
Tuesday:	3 P.M.–8 P.M. = 5 hours	
	8:30 P.M.–11 P.M. = 2.5 hours	
Wednesday:	7 A.M.–3 P.M. = 8 hours	
	3 P.M.–11 P.M. = 8 hours	

$(4.33 + 2.67 + 8) \times \$5.58 = \$83.70$
$(5 + 2.5 + 8) \times \$6.00 = \$93.00$

$\$83.70 + \$93.00 = \$176.70$

12. **(A)** $50 \times 20 = 1{,}000$ mg

13. **(B)** 1 marble : 37 = x marbles : 300
$37x = 300$
$x = 8.1 = 8$ marbles

14. **(B)** Interest = \$500
Rate = 8%
Time = 5 years
$P = x$

$I = PRT$
$500 = (P)(0.08)(5)$
$\$1{,}250 = P$

15. **(B)**

$$\frac{1}{3}(\$3,500) = \$1,167$$

$$\frac{1}{5}(\$3,500) = \$700$$

$$\frac{1}{4}(\$3,500) = \$875$$

$$\$3,500 - \$1,167 - \$700 - \$875 = \$758$$

16. **(D)** Interest = Principle × Rate × Time

$I = PRT$

$I = (750)(0.15)(2.17)$

$I = \$244.125 = \$244.13$

17. **(B)**

$$\frac{1}{6} = 17\%$$

17% of 89 students = 15.13 = 15 students
15% of 89 students = 13.35 = 13 students

$15 - 13 = 2$

18. **(B)** Graduate student #1 : 6 data sets/hour × 8 hours = 48 data sets
Graduate student #2 : 4.5 data sets/hour
Graduate student #1 + Graduate student #2 = 6 + 4.5 = 10.5 data sets/hour

854 data sets − 48 data sets = 806 data sets ÷ 10.5 data sets/hour = 77 hours

77 hours + 8 hours = 85 total hours

19. **(A)** Child 1 = 5 years old
Child 2 = 5 + 5 = 10 years old
Child 3 = 30 − 15 = 15 years old
Child 4 = 10 × 2 = 20 years old
Child 5 = 30 years old

20. **(A)** Jaw Lockers = \$2.50/lb
Sour Cherries = \$3.00/.5 lb = \$6.00/lb
Orange Blitzes = \$1.50/lb
Goofy Gum = \$.75/lb

$$\underline{(\$2.50 + \$6.00 + \$1.50 + \$.75)} =$$

$$\frac{\$10.75}{4} = \$2.69$$

21. **(A)** 34% of $3,514 = (0.34)(3,514) = $1,194.76
$3,514 − $1,194.76 − $150 = $2,169.24

22. **(D)**

23. **(A)**

24. **(A)**
$\angle D = 4x$
$\angle E = 2.5x$
$\angle F = x$

$4x + 2.5x + x = 180$
$7.5x = 180$
$x = 24°$
$4x = 96°$
$2.5x = 60°$

25. **(C)** $298.60 − $157.65 = $140.95 increase

$\dfrac{140.95}{157.65} = 0.894 = 89.4\%$

26. **(D)** x = ounces of dried fruit to be added mixture
$5 + x$ = total ounces of dried fruit in mixture
$8 + 6 + 4 + 5 + x$ = total weight of trail mix

Total ounces of dried fruit = 25% of total weight of trail mix
$5 + x = 0.25(8 + 6 + 4 + 5 + x)$
$5 + x = 0.25(23 + x)$
$20 + 4x = 1(23 + x)$
$3x = 3$
$x = 1$

27. **(C)** $\dfrac{\text{Desired} \times \text{Volume}}{\text{Available}}$ = mL per dose

$\dfrac{45 \text{ meq} \times 20 \text{ mL}}{30 \text{ meq}} = 30 \text{ mL} = 30$ mL/dose

28. **(A)** Increase = 350 mg
x = percentage of increase

What percent of 300 mg is 350 mg?
$300x = 350$
$x = 1.1666 = 1.17 = 117\%$ increase

29. **(C)** $(0.33 \times 596) + (0.20 \times 596) + (0.43 \times 596) = 197 + 119 + 256$
= 572 blankets distributed
596 − 572 = 24 blankets left in central supply

$$\frac{24}{596} = 4\% = 0.04 = \frac{1}{25}$$

30. **(C)** Original price = $146.25
Selling price = $1,162.50
$1,162.50 − $146.25 = $1,016.25

31. **(C)** $a^2 + b^2 = c^2$
$a^2 + 12^2 = 20^2$
$a^2 + 144 = 400$
$a^2 = 256$
$a = \sqrt{256}$
$a = 16$ feet

32. **(A)** $(75 \times \$.50) + (250 \times \$.25) + (150 \times \$.60) + (150 \times \$.15)$
$= \$37.50 + \$62.50 + \$90.00 + \$22.50$
$= \$212.50$

33. **(D)** Selling price − Purchase price = $148 − $20 = $128 overall profit
Profit/sandal = $8.50

$$\frac{128}{8.50} = 15.05 = 15 \text{ pairs of sandals}$$

34. **(C)**

35. **(B)** 1 tablet : 125 mg = x tablets : 1000 mg
$125 x = 1000$
$x = 8$ tablets

36. **(D)**

37. **(A)** $$\frac{60 \text{ mg}}{1 \text{ gr}} = \frac{x}{10 \text{ gr}}$$

$$60 \text{ mg} \times 10 \text{ gr} = x \times 1 \text{ gr}$$

$$\frac{60 \text{ mg} \times 10 \text{ gr}}{1 \text{ gr}} = \frac{x \times 1 \text{ gr}}{1 \text{ gr}}$$

$$x = 600 \text{ mg}$$

$$\frac{x}{600 \text{ mg}} = \frac{1 \text{ tablet}}{600 \text{ mg}}$$

$$x = 600 \text{ mg (1 tablet)}$$

38. **(A)**

39. **(B)**

$$\frac{78+84+56+96+78+85+85+95+0+73}{10} =$$

$$\frac{730}{10} = 73$$

40. **(A)**

41. **(C)**

42. **(C)** Selling price – Original cost – Refurbishing cost = Profit
$65,000 – $35,000 – $20,000 = $10,000

43. **(A)** x = hours
1 hour : 85 miles = x hours : 400 miles
$$86x = 400$$
$$x = 4.7 \text{ hours} = 4 \text{ hours } 42 \text{ minutes}$$

44. **(A)**

45. **(B)**

46. **(A)** $(10 \cdot \$15) + (5 \cdot \$7.50) + (18 \cdot \$4) +$
$(10 \cdot \$1.50) + (3 \cdot \$8.40)$
= $150 + $37.50 + $72 + $25 + $25.20
= $299.70

47. **(C)**
Magazine A = $458 – $13.74 = $444.26
Magazine B = $450 – $9.00 = $441
Magazine C = $480 – $24.00 = $456
Magazine D = $440

48. **(D)**

49. **(D)**

50. **(C)** x = total number of pencils in box

$\frac{1}{4}x$ = number of black pencils in box

$\frac{3}{8}x$ = number of red pencils in box

16 = number of yellow pencils in box

$$0.25x + 0.375x + 16 = x$$
$$0.625x + 16 = x$$
$$16 = 0.375x$$
$$42.875 = x = 43 \text{ pencils}$$

Answer Sheet
VERBAL ABILITY TEST

Verbal Ability

1 Ⓐ Ⓑ Ⓒ Ⓓ
2 Ⓐ Ⓑ Ⓒ Ⓓ
3 Ⓐ Ⓑ Ⓒ Ⓓ
4 Ⓐ Ⓑ Ⓒ Ⓓ
5 Ⓐ Ⓑ Ⓒ Ⓓ
6 Ⓐ Ⓑ Ⓒ Ⓓ
7 Ⓐ Ⓑ Ⓒ Ⓓ
8 Ⓐ Ⓑ Ⓒ Ⓓ
9 Ⓐ Ⓑ Ⓒ Ⓓ
10 Ⓐ Ⓑ Ⓒ Ⓓ
11 Ⓐ Ⓑ Ⓒ Ⓓ
12 Ⓐ Ⓑ Ⓒ Ⓓ
13 Ⓐ Ⓑ Ⓒ Ⓓ
14 Ⓐ Ⓑ Ⓒ Ⓓ
15 Ⓐ Ⓑ Ⓒ Ⓓ
16 Ⓐ Ⓑ Ⓒ Ⓓ
17 Ⓐ Ⓑ Ⓒ Ⓓ

18 Ⓐ Ⓑ Ⓒ Ⓓ
19 Ⓐ Ⓑ Ⓒ Ⓓ
20 Ⓐ Ⓑ Ⓒ Ⓓ
21 Ⓐ Ⓑ Ⓒ Ⓓ
22 Ⓐ Ⓑ Ⓒ Ⓓ
23 Ⓐ Ⓑ Ⓒ Ⓓ
24 Ⓐ Ⓑ Ⓒ Ⓓ
25 Ⓐ Ⓑ Ⓒ Ⓓ
26 Ⓐ Ⓑ Ⓒ Ⓓ
27 Ⓐ Ⓑ Ⓒ Ⓓ
28 Ⓐ Ⓑ Ⓒ Ⓓ
29 Ⓐ Ⓑ Ⓒ Ⓓ
30 Ⓐ Ⓑ Ⓒ Ⓓ
31 Ⓐ Ⓑ Ⓒ Ⓓ
32 Ⓐ Ⓑ Ⓒ Ⓓ
33 Ⓐ Ⓑ Ⓒ Ⓓ
34 Ⓐ Ⓑ Ⓒ Ⓓ

35 Ⓐ Ⓑ Ⓒ Ⓓ
36 Ⓐ Ⓑ Ⓒ Ⓓ
37 Ⓐ Ⓑ Ⓒ Ⓓ
38 Ⓐ Ⓑ Ⓒ Ⓓ
39 Ⓐ Ⓑ Ⓒ Ⓓ
40 Ⓐ Ⓑ Ⓒ Ⓓ
41 Ⓐ Ⓑ Ⓒ Ⓓ
42 Ⓐ Ⓑ Ⓒ Ⓓ
43 Ⓐ Ⓑ Ⓒ Ⓓ
44 Ⓐ Ⓑ Ⓒ Ⓓ
45 Ⓐ Ⓑ Ⓒ Ⓓ
46 Ⓐ Ⓑ Ⓒ Ⓓ
47 Ⓐ Ⓑ Ⓒ Ⓓ
48 Ⓐ Ⓑ Ⓒ Ⓓ
49 Ⓐ Ⓑ Ⓒ Ⓓ
50 Ⓐ Ⓑ Ⓒ Ⓓ

Answer Sheet

Verbal Ability Test

50 Test Items: TIME: 50 MINUTES

Directions: For each of the paired words, select the answer (A, B, C, or D) that best matches the paired words. Record your answers on the answer sheet on page 269.

1. DENTIST : TEETH ::
   DERMATOLOGIST :

   (A) DISEASE
   (B) BONES
   (C) SKIN
   (D) MUSCLES

2. BLANKET : MATTRESS ::

   (A) GRASS : GROUND
   (B) TIRE : PAVEMENT
   (C) LEAF : TREE
   (D) SHOE : SOCK

3. TROUT : FISH :: BULL :

   (A) SNAKE
   (B) DOG
   (C) COW
   (D) HIDE

4. GOOD : SWEET ::

   (A) BOY : GIRL
   (B) FOOD : VEGETABLE
   (C) NIGHT : DAY
   (D) BAD : SOUR

5. GAINES: *BLUE BOY* ::

   (A) LOSSES : *BASEBALL*
   (B) INCISIVE : *AORTA*
   (C) MICHELANGELO : *DAVID*
   (D) CAMUS : *MONK*

6. ATROPHY : DEGENERATE ::
   CHICANERY :

   (A) MEXICO
   (B) FLIGHT
   (C) TRICKERY
   (D) SICKLY

7. PROPERTY : VANDAL ::

   (A) BUILDING : POLICE
   (B) RELIGIOUS IMAGES :
       ICONOCLAST
   (C) UNDULATE : FLUCTUATE
   (D) WRATH : ANGRY

8. CIVIL WAR : HARPER'S FERRY ::

   (A) FRENCH REVOLUTION : BASTILLE
   (B) WORLD WAR I : VERSAILLES
   (C) KOREAN WAR : PANMUNJOM
   (D) WORLD WAR II : YALTA

9. DIMINUENDO : CRESCENDO ::
   ANDANTE :

   (A) SONATA
   (B) ALTO
   (C) VERDI
   (D) PRESTO

10. BEAR : FOX ::

    (A) BOVINE : CERVINE
    (B) PHYLUM : KINGDOM
    (C) EOCENE : PLIOCENE
    (D) URSINE : VULPINE

11. JOHN WAYNE : *THE COWBOYS* ::
    HARRISON FORD :

    (A) *IN HARM'S WAY*
    (B) *THE RAINMAKER*
    (C) *INDIANA JONES*
    (D) *THE KING AND I*

12. ABROGATE : NULLIFY ::

    (A) DELAY : RETARD
    (B) MAR : HEAL
    (C) HARDEN : INDULGE
    (D) APPLY : NEGLECT

13. ZANY : ZEST :: ZIP :

(A) JOIN
(B) FLEXIBLE
(C) ZOOM
(D) FAST

14. NEW MEXICO : "LAND OF ENCHANTMENT" ::

(A) TEXAS : "OIL"
(B) ILLINOIS : "LAND OF LINCOLN"
(C) WYOMING : "COWBOYS"
(D) ARIZONA : "LAND OF THE GREAT CANYON"

15. BOY : GIRL ::

(A) TALL : SHORT
(B) STRONG : WEAK
(C) BLUE : PINK
(D) FOOTBALL : GOLF

16. UGLY : APPALLING :: TURN OFF :

(A) UMBRAGE
(B) TALENTED
(C) DISGUST
(D) READY

17. DIFFUSE : COMPACT ::

(A) ASSUME : CONCLUDE
(B) AGREE : CONCUR
(C) COSTLY : DEAR
(D) FEEL : DOUBT

18. 150 : 450 ::

(A) 100 : 300
(B) 50 : 75
(C) 200 : 400
(D) 375 : 475

19. FIREMAN : AX :: POLICE OFFICER :

(A) BADGE
(B) GUN
(C) SIREN
(D) RADIO

20. SISTINE CHAPEL : ROME :: NOTRE DAME :

(A) FLORENCE
(B) PARIS
(C) PITTSBURGH
(D) BERLIN

21. TURNCOAT : TRAITOR :: WAX :

(A) WANE
(B) SHRINK
(C) INCREASE
(D) ABATE

22. BOTANIST : PLANTS :: HERPETOLOGIST :

(A) HERBS
(B) AMPHIBIANS
(C) FELINES
(D) FOWL

23. IMPUDENT : INCEPTION ::

(A) SAUCY : OUTSET
(B) IMMODERATE : DEDUCE
(C) NATURAL : NATIVE
(D) REFRACTORY : COMPULSION

24. PURBLIND : DIMSIGHTED :: RESCIND :

(A) REVOKE
(B) LUSTFUL
(C) DECENT
(D) CENSURE

25. ALERT : LETHARGIC ::

(A) LACONIC : VERBOSE
(B) MALEFACTOR : CRIMINAL
(C) LIMPID : LIPID
(D) SCOURGE : WHIP

26. SCINTILLA : REATA ::

(A) WISE : SAGE
(B) JOT : LARIAT
(C) REPROVE : REPRIMAND
(D) MATURE : VENILE

27. PULMONARY : LUNGS ::

    (A) RENAL : HEART
    (B) PALEO : LIFE
    (C) HEPATIC : LIVER
    (D) MUSCULAR : TISSUES

28. ABEYANCE : SUSTENANCE :: ASSIMILATE :

    (A) ABSORB
    (B) INTEGRATE
    (C) GENUINE
    (D) DISGORGE

29. CRYPTIC : HIDDEN ::

    (A) COULEE : GULCH
    (B) FRUSTRATE : SHORTCOME
    (C) MENTAL : VERIFY
    (D) GUILTY : CHURLISH

30. INCUBUS : NIGHTMARE :: BURDEN :

    (A) INDOLENT
    (B) PACK
    (C) CURSE
    (D) PLACID

31. DECEPTIVE : TRUE :: RICH :

    (A) FALSEHOOD
    (B) REFUTE
    (C) BLESSING
    (D) INDIGENT

32. TRIESTE : HUNGARY ::

    (A) BREST : FRANCE
    (B) VARNA : TURKEY
    (C) VENICE : DENMARK
    (D) REGA : AUSTRIA

33. NOVEMBER 22, 1963 : APRIL 5, 1865 ::

    (A) WASHINGTON : NIXON
    (B) TRUMAN : ROOSEVELT
    (C) JACKSON : JEFFERSON
    (D) KENNEDY : LINCOLN

34. $\frac{1}{2} : 0.5 :: \frac{7}{8} :$

    (A) 0.9
    (B) 0.875
    (C) 0.4375
    (D) 1.14

35. SAW : VERB :: BOY :

    (A) PERSONAL PRONOUN
    (B) NOUN
    (C) ADJECTIVE
    (D) CONJUNCTION

36. SUN : MERCURY ::

    (A) SUN : SATURN
    (B) SUN : EARTH
    (C) SUN : NEPTUNE
    (D) SUN : VENUS

37. INDEPENDENCE : SANTA FE TRAIL :: FT. BRIDGER :

    (A) OREGON TRAIL
    (B) CIMARRON CUTOFF
    (C) OLD SPANISH TRAIL
    (D) CUMBERLAND ROAD

38. FLOCK : SHEEP :: SHOAL :

    (A) GEESE
    (B) FISH
    (C) MICE
    (D) DUCKS

39. CHEYENNE : WYOMING :: DENVER :

    (A) UTAH
    (B) TEXAS
    (C) NEBRASKA
    (D) COLORADO

40. THERMOMETER : TEMPERATURE :: SPHYGMOMANOMETER :

    (A) HEART RATE
    (B) BLOOD PRESSURE
    (C) PULSE
    (D) RESPIRATIONS

41. X : TEN :: C :

    (A) ONE HUNDRED
    (B) TEN
    (C) ONE THOUSAND
    (D) ONE

42. DUMAS : *THE THREE MUSKETEERS* ::
DICKENS :

   (A) *OLIVER TWIST*
   (B) *SISTER CARRIE*
   (C) *AS I LAY DYING*
   (D) *MADAME BOVARY*

43. CRAZY HORSE : SIOUX :: QUANAH
PARKER :

   (A) MOHAWK
   (B) COMANCHE
   (C) APACHE
   (D) CROW

44. DECEMBER 25 : APRIL 1 ::

   (A) ARBOR DAY : MEMORIAL DAY
   (B) COLUMBUS DAY : LABOR DAY
   (C) CHRISTMAS DAY : APRIL FOOL'S
   DAY
   (D) PRESIDENT'S DAY : VALENTINE'S
   DAY

45. STERILE : FERTILE :: UNFRUITFUL :

   (A) STAID
   (B) TERSE
   (C) SALUBRIOUS
   (D) FECUND

46. DEONTOLOGY : ETHICS ::
HISTOLOGY :

   (A) FOSSILS
   (B) LIVING TISSUES
   (C) REVERED PERSONS
   (D) ANIMALS

47. PEARY : AMERICAN :: AMUNDSON :

   (A) SPANISH
   (B) ENGLISH
   (C) NORWEGIAN
   (D) FRENCH

48. BISMARCK : GERMANY ::

   (A) WHITNEY : AMERICA
   (B) GARIBALDI : ENGLAND
   (C) PIZARRO : ITALY
   (D) O'HIGGINS : CHILE

49. CUBISM : FRANCE ::

   (A) FUTURISM : ITALY
   (B) ENGRAVING : AMERICA
   (C) SURREALISM : CHINA
   (D) FAUVISM : BRAZIL

50. WILDER : *OUR TOWN* :: WILLIAMS :

   (A) *LEAVES OF GRASS*
   (B) *CAT ON A HOT TIN ROOF*
   (C) *THE COLOR PURPLE*
   (D) *THE HOBBIT*

STOP

If there is still time remaining, you may review your answers.

VERBAL ABILITY TEST ANSWER KEY

1. **(C)** A dentist specializes in the care of teeth. A dermatologist specializes in the care of skin.

2. **(A)** A blanket covers a bed. Grass covers the ground.

3. **(A)** Trout is a type of fish. A bull snake is a type of snake.

4. **(D)** Good and bad are antonyms, as are sweet and sour.

5. **(C)** Gaines painted the *Blue Boy*. Michelangelo sculpted *David*.

6. **(C)** Atrophy and degenerate are synonyms, as are chicanery and trickery.

7. **(B)** A vandal destroys property. An iconoclast destroys religious images.

8. **(A)** The first battle of the Civil War was fought at Harper's Ferry. The first battle of the French Revolution was fought at the Bastille.

9. **(D)** Diminuendo and crescendo are antonyms, as are andante and presto. All are musical terms.

10. **(D)** The adjective form of bear is ursine. The adjective form of fox is vulpine.

11. **(C)** The actor, John Wayne, starred in *The Cowboys*. The actor, Harrison Ford, starred in *Indiana Jones*.

12. **(A)** Abrogate and nullify are synonyms, as are delay and retard.

13. **(C)** All of the words begin with the letter *Z*.

14. **(B)** "Land of Lincoln" is inscribed on Illinois license plates. "Land of Enchantment" is inscribed on New Mexico license plates.

15. **(C)** Blue is typically considered a boy's color, whereas pink is typically considered a girl's color.

16. **(C)** Ugly and appalling are synonyms, as are turn off and disgust.

17. **(D)** Diffuse and compact are antonyms, as are feel and doubt.

18. **(A)** Four hundred fifty is three times greater than one hundred fifty. Three hundred is three times greater than one hundred.

19. **(B)** An ax is a hand tool for a fireman. A gun is a hand tool for a police officer.

Verbal Ability Test

20. **(B)** The Sistine Chapel is located in Rome. Notre Dame is located in Paris.

21. **(C)** Turncoat and traitor are synonyms, as are wax and increase.

22. **(B)** A botanist works with plants. A herpetologist works with amphibians.

23. **(A)** Impudent and saucy are synonyms, as are inception and outset.

24. **(A)** Purblind and dimsighted are synonyms, as are rescind and revoke.

25. **(A)** Alert and lethargic are antonyms, as are laconic and verbose.

26. **(B)** Scintilla and jot are synonyms, as are reata and lariat.

27. **(C)** The term *pulmonary* refers to the lungs. The term *hepatic* refers to the liver.

28. **(D)** Abeyance and sustenance are antonyms, as are assimilate and disgorge.

29. **(A)** Cryptic and hidden are synonyms, as are coulee and gulch.

30. **(B)** Incubus and nightmare are synonyms, as are burden and pack.

31. **(D)** Deceptive and true are antonyms, as are rich and indigent.

32. **(A)** The city of Trieste is in Hungary. The city of Brest is in France.

33. **(D)** President Kennedy was assassinated on November 22, 1963. President Lincoln was assassinated on April 5, 1865.

34. **(B)** One half is written both as a fraction and as a decimal. Seven-eighths is also written as a fraction and as a decimal.

35. **(B)** The word *saw* is a verb. The word *boy* is a noun.

36. **(D)** Mercury is the planet closest to the sun. Venus is the only other planet closer to the sun than Earth.

37. **(A)** The Santa Fe Trail began in Independence, Missouri. The Oregon Trail began at Ft. Bridger.

38. **(B)** A group of sheep is called a flock of sheep. A group of fish is called a shoal of fish.

39. **(D)** Cheyenne is the capital of the state of Wyoming. Denver is the capital of the state of Colorado.

40. **(B)** A thermometer is used to determine temperature. A sphygmomanometer is used to determine blood pressure.

41. **(A)** The number ten in Roman numerals is X. One hundred in Roman numerals is C.

42. **(A)** Dumas wrote the literary piece *The Three Musketeers*. Dickens wrote *Oliver Twist*.

43. **(B)** Crazy Horse was a Sioux chief. Quanah Parker was a Comanche chief.

44. **(C)** Christmas day is on December 25. April Fool's day is on April 1.

45. **(D)** Sterile and fertile are antonyms, as are unfruitful and fecund. Sterile and unfruitful are synonyms, as are fertile and fecund.

46. **(B)** Deontology is the study of ethics. Histology is the study of living tissues.

47. **(C)** Peary was an American. He was the first to reach the North Pole. Amundsen was a Norwegian. He was the first to reach the South Pole.

48. **(D)** Bismarck is considered the unifier of Germany. O'Higgins is considered the unifier of Chile.

49. **(A)** The art style, cubism, developed in France. The art style, futurism, developed in Italy.

50. **(B)** Thornton Wilder wrote *Our Town*. Tennessee Williams wrote *Cat on a Hot Tin Roof*.

Verbal Ability Test

Answer Sheet
SCIENCE TEST

Science

1 (A) (B) (C) (D)
2 (A) (B) (C) (D)
3 (A) (B) (C) (D)
4 (A) (B) (C) (D)
5 (A) (B) (C) (D)
6 (A) (B) (C) (D)
7 (A) (B) (C) (D)
8 (A) (B) (C) (D)
9 (A) (B) (C) (D)
10 (A) (B) (C) (D)
11 (A) (B) (C) (D)
12 (A) (B) (C) (D)
13 (A) (B) (C) (D)
14 (A) (B) (C) (D)
15 (A) (B) (C) (D)
16 (A) (B) (C) (D)
17 (A) (B) (C) (D)

18 (A) (B) (C) (D)
19 (A) (B) (C) (D)
20 (A) (B) (C) (D)
21 (A) (B) (C) (D)
22 (A) (B) (C) (D)
23 (A) (B) (C) (D)
24 (A) (B) (C) (D)
25 (A) (B) (C) (D)
26 (A) (B) (C) (D)
27 (A) (B) (C) (D)
28 (A) (B) (C) (D)
29 (A) (B) (C) (D)
30 (A) (B) (C) (D)
31 (A) (B) (C) (D)
32 (A) (B) (C) (D)
33 (A) (B) (C) (D)
34 (A) (B) (C) (D)

35 (A) (B) (C) (D)
36 (A) (B) (C) (D)
37 (A) (B) (C) (D)
38 (A) (B) (C) (D)
39 (A) (B) (C) (D)
40 (A) (B) (C) (D)
41 (A) (B) (C) (D)
42 (A) (B) (C) (D)
43 (A) (B) (C) (D)
44 (A) (B) (C) (D)
45 (A) (B) (C) (D)
46 (A) (B) (C) (D)
47 (A) (B) (C) (D)
48 (A) (B) (C) (D)
49 (A) (B) (C) (D)
50 (A) (B) (C) (D)

Science Test

50 Test Items: TIME: 90 MINUTES

Directions: Read and answer the following questions. Record your answers on the answer sheet on page 279. Note that many of these science questions call upon the reader's skills in reading comprehension as well as basic knowledge of science. Please refer to the Science Review section, Chapter Six, and the Reading Comprehension areas in Chapter Four in order to prepare to answer these questions.

Biology, Zoology, and Microbiology

Living things must be able to perform certain functions in order to survive. In a very broad sense, functions could be categorized as movement, taking in from the environment, putting out to the environment, passing on one's makeup, and interior communication.

With this information in mind, respond to questions 1–16.

1. According to this short description, which of the following are overall functions of living things?

   (A) circulation, respiration, elimination
   (B) anthropomorphism, cancellation
   (C) representation, amelioration, traction
   (D) none of the above

2. Which of the following diseases is caused by an organism commonly transmitted through the bite of a mosquito?

   (A) influenza
   (B) whooping cough
   (C) polio
   (D) malaria

3. Which of the following types of tissues grows most rapidly?

   (A) bone
   (B) epithelial
   (C) nervous
   (D) skeletal muscle

4. White blood cell deficiency would predispose a living creature to problems with

   (A) bleeding.
   (B) blood clotting.
   (C) fatigue.
   (D) infection.

5. Red blood cell deficiency would predispose a living creature to problems with

   (A) bleeding.
   (B) fatigue.
   (C) infection.
   (D) joint swelling.

6. Platelet deficiency would predispose a living creature to problems with

   (A) bleeding.
   (B) fatigue.
   (C) infection.
   (D) forgetfulness.

7. Which type of metabolism is preferred by humans and other higher level creatures?

   (A) aerobic
   (B) anaerobic
   (C) nutrient
   (D) biodegradable

8. Which of the following elements are routinely measured with a blood test as part of hospitalization or in a routine examination?

   (A) corpuscular volume
   (B) lactic acid and vitamin C
   (C) ammonia and phosphokinase
   (D) sodium and potassium

9. Which of the following is an anion?

   (A) sodium
   (B) potassium
   (C) chloride
   (D) magnesium

10. Which of the following is the preferred pH range in mammals?

    (A) 3 to 4
    (B) approximately 10
    (C) in the mid-7 region
    (D) 5.2 to 6.1

11. Connective tissue would be most likely to appear in

    (A) the semicircular canals of the ear.
    (B) the brain.
    (C) the nose.
    (D) muscle.

12. Which of the following are made up of a type of connective tissue?

    (A) epithelial linings
    (B) fatty tissues
    (C) reproductive cells, such as eggs and sperm
    (D) nerves

13. In which areas in mammals is muscle tissue located?

    (A) the liver and pancreas
    (B) the heart and gastrointestinal tract
    (C) the kidney and brain
    (D) the teeth and interior of the eyeball

14. Which of the following is a type of nervous tissue?

    (A) sensory
    (B) motor
    (C) peripheral
    (D) all the above

15. Which of the following would be a particularly dangerous thing to do for the person with a moderately ineffective immune system?

    (A) eating canned foods or shopping in public places
    (B) gardening or cleaning the fish tank
    (C) oversleeping
    (D) driving a car

16. Which of the following are accurate statements?

    (A) All members of the animal kingdom have GI tracts.
    (B) Food absorbed into the bloodstream from the GI tract must consist of more complex substances than those taken into the mouth. Enzymes accomplish this.
    (C) Byproducts of nutrient elements that dwell too long in the lower areas of the GI tract will be very liquid and will result in diarrhea.
    (D) In the case of vertebrates, food taken in need not be completely clean, since the hydrochloric acid of the stomach will kill many germs.

Science Test

When dealing with anatomic descriptions in a nursing context, a reference to the right side always means the patient's right side, rather than the examiner's right side. Proximal means near to the center of the body and distal means farther away. Anterior means at the front and posterior at the back. Abduction involves moving a limb away from the center of the body and adduction means moving toward. Flexion is bending and extension is straightening.

With these terms in mind, accurately complete questions 17–20.

17. The wrist is _____ to the elbow.

    (A) anterior
    (B) posterior
    (C) proximal
    (D) distal

18. The airway is _____ to the food tube, or esophagus.

    (A) anterior
    (B) posterior
    (C) proximal
    (D) distal

19. When standing upright, the knees are

    (A) flexed.
    (B) extended.
    (C) obtuse.
    (D) at a 90° angle.

20. Considering the anatomy of the respiratory system, down which side of the lung's bronchi (airway) would a suction tube be likely to pass?

    (A) left
    (B) right
    (C) middle
    (D) posterior

Nearsightedness involves the ability to see things that are closer to the eyes, whereas farsightedness involves adequate distance vision but poor close-up vision. Numbers are used to describe relative clarity of vision. If a person has 20/20 vision, then what the individual sees at 20 feet away is what an average person with normal vision would see 20 feet from an object. If the person has 20/10 vision, this is better than average. What is seen at 20 feet away by this individual is what an average person would have to be 10 feet away from to see clearly.

With this distinction in mind, respond to questions 21 and 22.

21. Your friend is told he has 20/200 vision. This level of vision would be

   (A) excellent.
   (B) average.
   (C) poor.
   (D) none of the above.

22. Another friend is told she is farsighted. In which situation would you expect this person to squint or to have the most trouble seeing clearly?

   (A) when watching television from her easy chair
   (B) when scanning the horizon to spot the tornado that is in the area
   (C) when trying to read the newspaper
   (D) after dark at any distance

Refer to Chapter Six for questions 23–26.

23. Within the nervous system of living things, transmission of impulses between nerve cells happens by

   (A) electrical discharge.
   (B) transmitter substances.
   (C) regeneration.
   (D) degeneration.

24. Which of the following are signs of inflammation?

   (A) pallor, pulselessness
   (B) cool temperature, blue color
   (C) heat, redness
   (D) green discharge, no change in skin color

25. Which of the following are essential nutrients for humans?

    (A) fats, carbohydrate, proteins, and water
    (B) vitamins and minerals
    (C) all the above
    (D) none of the above

26. Which of the following are nutrient forms that may circulate through the bloodstream?

    (A) glucose, cholesterol, lipids, and amino acids
    (B) starches, chyme, and protein
    (C) cellulose and complex carbohydrates
    (D) ammonia and bilirubin

Chemistry

Diffusion and osmosis are two methods by which substances pass from one body compartment to another. Diffusion occurs as substances follow a natural tendency to spread out from their point of origin. Osmosis involves the tendency of substances to spread out, but in a different way. When substances must pass through a membrane, those that are able to dissolve into simple ions will pass through, along with liquid. With osmosis, the more complex substances, such as starch or protein molecules, will not pass through, but liquids will be drawn to their "complex" side of the membrane until concentrations are approximately equal.

With this description in mind, please respond to questions 27–30.

27. According to your understanding, which of the following reflects diffusion?

    (A) the combining of simple elements into complex compounds
    (B) the passage of liquids through a membrane, usually "drawn in" by complex molecules
    (C) the passage of substances in solution from an area of higher concentration to an area of lower concentration
    (D) the splitting of the atom

28. Which represents osmosis?

    (A) the combining of simple elements into complex compounds
    (B) the passage of liquids through a membrane, usually "drawn in" by complex molecules
    (C) the passage of substances in solution from an area of higher concentration to an area of lower concentration
    (D) the splitting of the atom

29. Which of the following types of atoms would be more likely to bond together to form a compound?

    (A) those of the same family
    (B) those with incomplete outer electron shells
    (C) heavy metals
    (D) radioactive substances

30. What is the relationship between a solution and a colloid?

    (A) One is thicker than the other.
    (B) One can pass in entirety through semipermeable membranes; the other can only attract liquids through a semipermeable membrane.
    (C) Both circulate through living beings.
    (D) All the above.

Genetics

All living organism inherit traits from parents. Traits contain encodes from the hereditary material known as deoxyribonucleic acid (DNA), which is composed of genes. DNA is formed from four chemical bases. These are repeated over and over again. The human being has three billion pairs of bases. The chemicals are specific in order and appearance. The order underlies all of life's diversity, clearly determining one organism from another. Gregor Mendel first discovered inherited characteristics, and that genetic makeup could be determined from these inherited characteristics. This is true for plants and animals as well. A person inherits one gene for a given characteristic, such as eye color, from one parent and one from the other parent.

Some genes are dominant and some are recessive. If a person inherits a dominant gene from one parent and a recessive gene from the other, the dominant gene will determine the trait. If two recessive genes are inherited, the recessive trait will be inherited. For example, if the gene for brown eyes is dominant, and the gene for blue eyes is recessive, the child has a one-in-one chance of having blue eyes if both parents have the recessive gene. See the chart below:

		Parent #1	
		BROWN (B)	blue (b)
	BROWN (B)	BB	Bb
Parent #2			
	blue (b)	bB	bb

According to your understanding of the laws of inheritance based on this material, respond to questions 31–33.

31. If a disease is in a recessive gene and both parents have the recessive gene, but not the disease, what are the odds that a baby will be born with the disease?

    (A) One in four (25%)
    (B) One in two (50%)
    (C) One in three (75%)
    (D) The child will be born with the disease (100%).

32. One parent has two dominant genes for ordinary skin tone; the other has the dominant gene and a recessive gene for wrinkled skin. What are the chances that a child will be born with the wrinkled skin characteristic?

    (A) 25%
    (B) 50%
    (C) 75%
    (D) The child will definitely *not* be born with a tendency to develop wrinkled skin (100%).

33. Using data from the previous case, if the couple has four children, how many would perhaps be likely to carry the recessive gene forward into other generations?

    (A) None
    (B) One
    (C) Two
    (D) Three

Since the inception of the Human Genome Project (HGP), scientists are studying and discovering more and more about the influence of genetics, inherited characteristics, and the behavior of human beings. In an advanced nature, more is studied and researched about DNA sequencing. DNA sequencing is utilized to search genetic variations and mutations that perhaps are vital in the development or progression of a particular disease. The HGP discovered that probably 20,500 human genes exist. This information provides the structure, organization, and function of the complete set of human genes.

The results from evaluating a study of one set of identical twins (both raised separately) reflect the relative influence of genetics or inherited characteristics as they relate to behavior: for example, relative levels of aggressive or passive tendencies, adult preferences for foods and beverages, preference in cars, and even the tendency to take risks. The selection of a mate is spectacularly different in twins. Apparently, tendencies to be attracted to the opposite sex are more a product of circumstance than inheritance.

In view of the main themes of the paragraph, select the best responses for questions 34–36.

34. Which of the following might be an accurate statement related to alcoholism and inheritance?

    (A) The tendency to drink alcohol too heavily is entirely dependent on genetic inheritance.
    (B) The tendency to become an alcoholic has nothing to do with inherited characteristics.
    (C) The tendency to become an alcoholic is probably a result of both nurture and nature.
    (D) There can be no inference about inheritance and alcoholism based on the paragraph presented.

35. Which of the following would be likely when two twins raised apart are brought together as adults?

    (A) They will have similar levels of intelligence because intelligence is determined by early childhood experience as well as genetic inheritance.
    (B) They will probably drive the same type of sports car.
    (C) They will have similar occupations.
    (D) All the above.

36. The nature versus nurture controversy, with twin studies as a prime method for making determinations, is important because

    (A) behavioral scientists and those trying to solve problems of humanity will have an easier time if they know what human characteristics are changeable; which ones are not patterned in from the time of birth.
    (B) cloning, or the making of identical creatures in order to preserve certain characteristics, is dependent on our investigating behaviors of twins.
    (C) twins possess extrasensory perception (ESP).
    (D) twins survive catastrophe, such as fires and earthquakes, better than others; scientists must discover why.

First Aid and Emergency Practices

37. You come upon a person who is waiting for the same bus you are. The person is sweating profusely, even on this crisp autumn day, and states, "I just don't feel well." Which of the following actions would involve the best judgment?

    (A) Consider that the person might have a fever or be contagious. Stay at least 2 or 3 feet away, but continue talking with him to determine any other symptoms.
    (B) Take his pulse, since he might be having a heart attack. Then direct him to go to the nearest hospital.
    (C) Since he looks quite unwell, and you aren't sure what is wrong, offer to run back to your house, get your car, and take him to the doctor or hospital.
    (D) Have him sit and try to relax. Call Emergency Medical Services.

    Triage involves making decisions, in an emergency situation in which resources are stretched, about those who are likely to survive the catastrophe and those who are very unlikely to survive. When triage decisions are made, the rescuing groups are able to concentrate their lifesaving resources on those who have some chance of survival. This does not mean that those triaged into the nonsurvivable category cannot survive. It only means that, for the duration of the crisis, and until reserves arrive, those with the highest likelihood of survival will need to be temporarily cared for first. The term *triage* is from a French word involving the number three. In simplified form, this means that casualties are sorted into three groups: those who probably will not survive, those who will survive and are capable of walking about and helping, and those who can survive but are not encouraged to be or are incapable of being ambulatory.

Based on the paragraph concerning triage, respond to questions 38–40.

38. Determine which of the following decisions made by the triage nurse is correct.

    (A) Placing the person with profuse bleeding into the nonsurvivable group
    (B) Placing the person with the splinted fractured arm into the category of those who are ambulatory and can help
    (C) Placing the wheezing person with extensive shrapnel wounds and third degree, full-thickness burns over 95% of the body into the survivable group
    (D) None of the choices provided is a correct decision.

39. A disaster has occurred in a major city. You are the triage nurse. Which of the following, provided the statement was truthful and accurate, would be an appropriate response to a family member who notices that her loved one, who is unconscious and has been placed in the nonsurvivable group, is not being cared for with the same diligence as another victim who has been placed in a survivable group of patients?

    (A) "Go back into the waiting area. This section is for patients and care-givers only. We'll call you later."
    (B) "What is your loved one's name? We are watching him for any signs of discomfort, but, with his injuries, he is perhaps going to have an uphill battle to survive. We are expecting the National Guard medics to arrive at any minute and will reevaluate his condition then. But he is quite seriously ill, so you may want to sit by him for awhile."
    (C) "He is in the nonsurvivable group. You may want to pray for him. Other health care personnel will arrive any time now, and we can reeval-uate his situation then, when we have more people and supplies."
    (D) "I'm not allowed to talk about his condition. The doctor is responsible for making decisions about care, so, if it seems to you that your loved one isn't being well cared for, you might want to try to find the physi-cian so that you can discuss this with him. Or, if you'd prefer, I can page him."

40. You are working as a nursing assistant in a big city emergency room with twenty separate stations for the treatment of patients. There are four resi-dents and six interns within the confines of the hospital on this night, all of whom are capable of performing ER functions. In addition, there is a staff of eight ER nurses, and there are two secretaries on duty. Which of the follow-ing situations would qualify as a triage situation?

    (A) There has been a two-car accident and the radio from a local ambulance announces that the four victims are headed your way.
    (B) An airplane taking off for Europe has traveled beyond the runway of the local international airport and a police call alerts you that this was a barely survivable crash.
    (C) A phone call alerts the staff that 25 conventioneers are apparently suffer-ing from food poisoning after eating at a local restaurant. Complaints include stomach cramps and headache. Some state that they feel they are going to pass out.
    (D) All the above.

General Science

Fahrenheit to Centigrade conversions involve working with formulas.
Convert questions 41–44 using the formula of

$$\frac{9}{5}C + 32 = F$$

41. If $C = 0°$, then

   (A) $F = 0°$.
   (B) $F = 100°$.
   (C) $F = 32°$.
   (D) $F = 64°$.

42. If $C = 36°$, then

   (A) $F = -2°$.
   (B) $F = 63°$.
   (C) $F = 347°$.
   (D) $F = 95°$.

43. If $F = 77°$, then

   (A) $C = 25°$.
   (B) $C = 45°$.
   (C) $C = -212°$.
   (D) $C = 81°$.

44. If $F = 98.6°$, then

   (A) $C = 100.0°$.
   (B) $C = 66.6°$.
   (C) $C = 37.0°$.
   (D) $C = 0°$.

Earthquakes arise, in part, as a result of large plates of the earth's crust slowly rotating and grinding past each other in the normal course of movement. Areas of the planet that lie above a section of plate that is likely to move are said to lie upon a fault line.

These plates may also move slightly about the surface of the earth. Looking at a map of Europe, Africa, and the Americas, one can almost visualize how these mighty continents once nested against each other. The borders of the continents resemble pieces of a puzzle that, if slightly rotated and fitted together, would provide an exact match in terms of outline.

Based on this passage, select the correct answers to questions 45–47.

45. Which of the following areas are most likely to lie along active fault lines?

 (A) New England
 (B) England
 (C) Japan
 (D) Antarctica

46. Which of the following has never been known to be predictive of a pending earthquake?

 (A) strange behavior of animals
 (B) seismic (vibration) monitoring of the ground
 (C) weather patterns
 (D) a slight rise or fall in the configuration of the ground along a fault line

47. Which would be most logical in protecting yourself in the midst of an earthquake?

 (A) You hide in a closet in the center of the house. If there are no closets, you hide in the fireplace.
 (B) You jump in the car and try to outrun the quake.
 (C) You get outside and away from all buildings. Get into a doorframe and brace yourself if there is no easy way to reach the street.
 (D) You go to the upper stories of your building so that you can be picked up by helicopter if the situation worsens. This will also allow you to see if a fault line is extending toward you.

Science and Research

Human beings are characterized by the ability to be self-aware and to perform complex cognitive operations, such as research. Research involves the ability to reason.

There are two major types of reasoning: inductive and deductive. With inductive reasoning, one moves from a series of specific facts to form a generalization. For example, one notices that plants on one side of a house grow more rapidly than those on the other. One might form a hypothesis, or working generalization, that there is something about the light, moisture, or air circulation conditions on the sides of the house that enhance or retard growth. One could then test this hypothesis through active experimentation.

In the case of deductive reasoning, one comes to the situation equipped with a set of rules or of generalizations. One then tests to see if circumstances of a given situation fit. This is the type of reasoning employed by the fictitious detective, Sherlock Holmes. For example, if one is aware that horses shy away from a large hat waved in their faces, and one discovers a horse that does not follow this rule, then one might conclude that the horse is blind or neurologically afflicted in some way, or has been trained to ignore large objects waved in the face. Research may be observational, in which the investigator observes but takes no active hand, and experimental, in which the investigator performs an active intervention and then observes results. Nursing research may be qualitative, in which the investigator typically studies small numbers of things intensively and without preformed conclusions, or quantitative, in which the investigator studies larger numbers. For example, observing patients entering a clinic for signs of nervousness would be observational and would seem to be qualitative. One is not sure in advance if one will see tremulousness, unusual speech patterns, pacing in front of the registration desk, voice changes, or other indications of nervousness. If one actually surveyed a large group, using a written questionnaire designed to elicit statements of relaxation or nervousness and then one instituted measures in the clinic designed to promote relaxation, measuring after-the-fact to detect change, then that would fall into the category of experimental research of a quantitative nature.

With this in mind, please answer questions 48–50.

48. Inductive reasoning results in

   (A) experiments.
   (B) formation of generalizations.
   (C) proving that generalizations are true.
   (D) intensive interviewing of research participants.

49. Which of the following is an example of hypothesis testing in scientific research?

    (A) speculating that stimuli produce responses
    (B) forming an opinion that women truck drivers can remain alert at the wheel longer than men
    (C) developmentally, observing whether children always develop their finer motor skills from the head downward
    (D) wondering, in a scientific journal, whether Florida natives are more likely to develop skin cancer than those who retired to Florida in old age

50. Which statement expresses a major difference between research-based conclusions and simple opinion?

    (A) Research is rigorous and involves techniques developed over centuries of using logic. It results in a strong likelihood that one's conclusions fit reality.
    (B) Opinion can be just as strong as more formal research, in that most of the research takes place in one's mind, so that, although not subject to scrutiny by others, the conclusions may be just as valid as those based on more formal research.
    (C) There is no real difference.
    (D) Research is subject to preformed bias; opinion is not.

STOP

If there is still time remaining, you may review your answers.

Science Test

SCIENCE TEST ANSWER KEY

1. **(A)** Living things engage in circulation, respiration, and elimination.

2. **(D)** Mosquitoes transmit malaria.

3. **(B)** Epithelial tissue grows most rapidly.

4. **(D)** White blood cells are involved with the immune response, so a deficiency could create a tendency to develop infection.

5. **(B)** Red blood cell deficiency is anemia, a disorder characterized by fatigue.

6. **(A)** Platelets are involved with the clotting process, so a deficit would be characterized by bleeding.

7. **(A)** Aerobic metabolism happens in the presence of plentiful supplies of oxygen during normal circumstances.

8. **(D)** This routine chemistry test involves these seven substances: sodium, potassium, chloride, carbon dioxide, urea nitrogen, creatinine, and glucose.

9. **(C)** Cations have a positive charge and go first in the naming of substances that form ions in solution. Anions have a negative charge and go second.

10. **(C)** Mammals prefer a serum pH range of 7.35 to 7.45.

11. **(C)** Cartilage, in the nose, is connective tissue.

12. **(B)** Fat is a type of connective tissue.

13. **(B)** The heart and gastrointestinal tract are made up of muscle tissue.

14. **(D)** Nervous tissues are of three types: peripheral, afferent (sensory), or efferent (motor).

15. **(B)** There are no particular dangers involved with sleeping or driving. Canned foods are typically safe. But the exotic microbes found in soil or fish tanks are dangerous to those with inferior immune responses.

16. **(D)** Vertebrates eat unclean food and the stomach's hydrochloric acid kills many germs.

17. **(D)** The wrist lies below, or distal to, the elbow.

18. **(A)** The airway is in front of, or anterior to, the esophagus.

19. **(A)** The knees are extended (180° angle) when standing.

20. **(B)** Since the right mainstem bronchus is straighter, a tube would pass down the right more easily.

21. **(C)** The person would only be able to see at 20 feet what a person with average eyesight could be standing 200 feet away and see.

22. **(C)** Farsightedness means that the person has no trouble seeing things that are far (as opposed to very close, such as reading material).

23. **(B)** Transmitter substances convey impulses.

24. **(C)** Inflamed areas are swollen, hot, red, painful, and unable to function in normal fashion.

25. **(C)** The essential nutrients are fats, carbohydrates, proteins, water, vitamins, and minerals.

26. **(A)** The simplest forms can circulate in the bloodstream. Choices B and C involve complex entities, and choice D is not a set of nutrient substances, but, rather, byproducts to be eliminated.

27. **(C)** Diffusion is passage from higher to lower concentration.

28. **(B)** Osmosis is passage toward complex molecules.

29. **(B)** Electron shells completely filled are satisfied and do not bond with other elements.

30. **(D)** All of the above. Colloids and solutions circulate; solutions are thinner and can pass through.

31. **(A)** If the letter *D* stands for dominant and the letter *r* stands for recessive, then each parent could contribute a Dr set. Neither parent could contribute an rr set, since then the disease would be evident in the parent with these two recessive genes. The four possibilities to be formed from the two *D*s and the two *r*s are DD, rr, Dr, and Dr. Only the rr situation will allow the child to exhibit active disease characteristics.

32. **(D)** If the letter *O* is the dominant gene for ordinary skin, and the letter *w* is the recessive gene for wrinkled skin, the combinations from the OO parent and the Ow parent become OO, OO, Ow, and Ow. Since, in no case, does ww emerge, the recessive trait cannot emerge in the form of wrinkled skin.

33. **(C)** Of the combinations produced (OO, OO, Ow, and Ow), the odds are that two out of the four children would carry the recessive gene.

34. **(C)** Nurture and nature may be involved in alcoholism.

35. **(D)** Intelligence and certain preference may be genetically influenced.

36. **(A)** Nature implies genetically determined and not necessarily changeable; nurture involves experience.

37. **(D)** Because a heart attack is a potentially nonsurvivable event, the symptomatic person should rest, decreasing stress on the heart, and the rescuer should quickly bring professionals to him.

38. **(B)** A person with an arm fracture may assist others.

39. **(B)** This conveys the total picture to the person, but with a sense of caring and kindness, and a suggestion of what course the family member might take.

40. **(B)** Knowing that very large aircraft fly transatlantic routes, one can surmise there will be more than 100 casualties. The other scenarios probably wouldn't threaten to overwhelm the personnel or material resources of this large emergency room.

41. **(C)** $0 + 32 = 32°$

42. **(D)** $\frac{9}{5}(36) + 32 = 95°$

43. **(A)** $\frac{9}{5}C + 32 = 77$

$$\frac{9}{5}C = 77 - 32$$

$$C = \frac{5}{9}(45) = 25°$$

44. **(C)** $\frac{9}{5}C + 32 = 98.6$

$$\frac{9}{5}C = 98.6 - 32$$

$$C = \frac{5}{9}(66.6)$$

$$C = 37.0°$$

45. **(C)** The only area known to have frequent earthquakes is Japan.

46. **(C)** Weather is the only phenomenon that arises above and is distinct from ground level.

47. **(C)** All other choices would expose one to injury from building collapse.

48. **(B)** Inductive moves from specific to general.

49. **(C)** This is the only choice that moves from a general rule to examination of specific cases. The researcher actually tests something.

50. **(A)** Research involves rigor and specialized techniques.

References

Czarnecki, L. (2011). Minerals and mineralogy. *http://www.hpwt.de/Mineral2e.htm.*

National Human Genome Research Instittue. (2008).*Genetic and Genomic Nursing: Competencies, Curricula Guidelines and Outcome Indicators.* (2nd ed.). *http://www.genome.gov/17517037.*

Junglen, L.M., Pestka, E.L., Clawson, M.L., & Fisher, S.D. (2008) Incorporating genetics and genomics into nursing practice: A demonstration. *The Online Journal of Issues in Nursing,* 13(3), DOI: 10.3912/OJIN.Vol13No03PPT02.

Kee, J., & Marshall, S. (2009). *Clinical calculations: With applications to general and specialty areas,* (6th ed.). Philadelphia: Saunders.

Mosby. (2011). *Mosby's Nursing Drug Reference* (24th ed.). St. Louis: Mosby.

Mussak, E. (2010). The passage of time. *http://www.whatithinkabout.com/the-passage-of-time/.*

Phillips, B. (1966). *Social Research: Strategy and Tactics.* The nature of simulation. New York: MacMillian.

Index

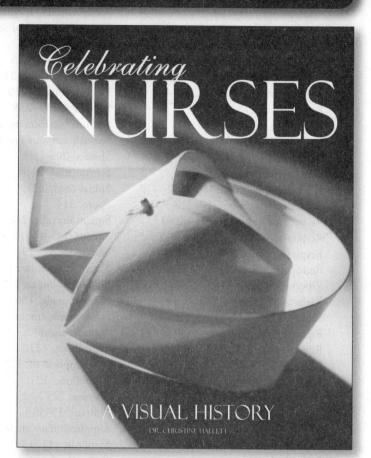
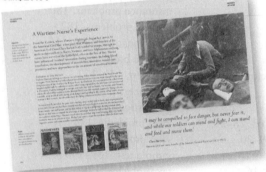
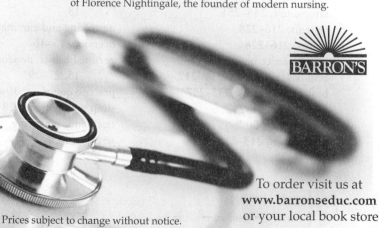

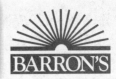
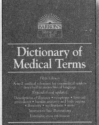
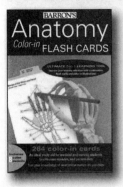
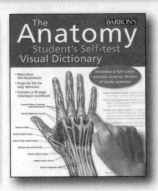
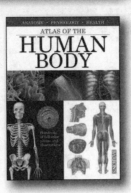
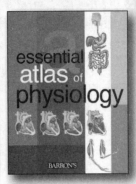
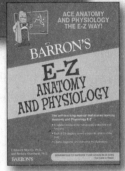

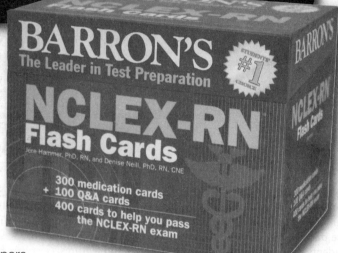
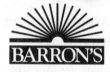
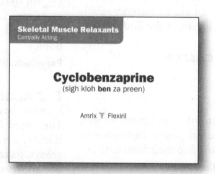
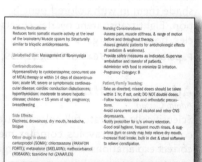
HILLSBORO PUBLIC LIBRARIES
Hillsboro, OR
Member of Washington County
COOPERATIVE LIBRARY SERVICES